GO FIND JOY

The Science of Calm:
Erasing Anxiety with Energy Therapy

MARK L. FOX
Foreword by: Dr. Pedram Shojai, The Urban Monk

Mark L. Fox-- 1st ed.
Chief Editor, Shannon Buritz
ISBN: 978-1-954757-59-2
Remarkable Press

The Publisher has strived to be as accurate and complete as possible in the creation of this book.

This book is not intended for use as a legal, business, accounting, or financial advice source. All readers are advised to seek the services of competent professionals in legal, business, accounting, and finance fields.

Like anything else in life, there are no guarantees of income or results in practical advice books. Readers are cautioned to rely on their judgment about their individual circumstances to act accordingly.

While all attempts have been made to verify information provided in this publication, the Publisher assumes no responsibility for errors, omissions, or contrary interpretation of the subject matter herein. Any perceived slights of specific persons, peoples, or organizations are unintentional.

CONTENTS

FOREWORD

The writing is on the wall. You've got to feel safe to heal and thrive. Our modern world is bombarding us with toxins, stressors, and artificial foods that make it hard to feel well.

All of this affects the nervous system, and the place we see this most is the vagus nerve.

I began seeking out vagus nerve stimulators for my clinics many years ago, and it was tough. The industry wasn't there, and the technology was big and clunky.

I knew the intrinsic value, but it was still easier to teach patients abdominal breathing vs wrestling with the bad gadgets we had.

For years, I've been playing with the new models and finally found one I loved. It was affordable and effective, and the inventor was involved in a number of clinical studies.

Here we had a rocket scientist, Space Shuttle Chief Engineer, who tinkered with the tech and created something amazing. He was humble about it and said "I don't know" a lot, which is an important stance in science.

A scientist he was and is.

Mark Fox is always exploring and working to better his projects, and it's been a delight working with him. He's genuinely interested in helping people, and I believe he's created a scalable solution that can do just that.

Finding joy is much easier when we feel safe. It's possible when the bullets aren't flying.

That's the power of the vagus nerve and what Mark has been working on is revolutionary.

This book will help you.

Dr. Pedram Shojai
The Urban Monk

INTRODUCTION

If you're like most people with anxiety, you're struggling with all of the mental anguish that comes with it. You've tried the medication; maybe it worked for a little while, or perhaps it didn't. Maybe the side effects were worse than the original issue. You've seen the six o'clock news. You know how those commercials sound. The list of "possible side effects" is like something out of a horror movie.

What you really want—what you *deserve*—is to find joy in your life again. Not a temporary high or a distraction, but real, lasting joy. Freedom from the pain. Freedom from the pills. Freedom from the side effects that leave you feeling like a shell of yourself. And you want a solution that's not tied to an office visit or a prescription bottle.

You're not alone. Anxiety is the number one ailment in the world. And it's not your fault that you haven't found something that works yet. Most people haven't heard of Pulsed Electromagnetic Field therapy—PEMF—because their doctors likely haven't either. Or if they have, they're too scared to step outside the lines drawn by the American Medical Association. It's not necessarily their fault. Most of them aren't trained in anything but conventional medicine. They're not being taught alternatives. They're being handed drug reps and expensive vacations disguised as "continuing education."

You don't see energy therapy commercials on TV because drug companies own the airwaves. Turn on the news any time of day, and what do you see? Drug ads. Everywhere. Pfizer, Eli Lilly, all of them. Did you know that pharmaceutical companies fund 75% of the FDA's research budget? That's not a conspiracy theory. That's a business model. And it's working for them.

But here's the part that matters to you: energy therapy, such as PEMF, isn't part of that system. It doesn't have billion-dollar ad budgets or lobbyists in Washington. What it *does* have is results backed by science and, more importantly, by stories. Stories from people who found their joy again. People like you.

If you're skeptical, I understand. After 20 years of trying everything under the sun, from pills and patches to therapy and implants, you've earned the right to be cautious. Most people who come to me are already on their twelfth medication. Some are on their second surgery. A few have mechanical implants, nerve blockers, spinal stimulators, and still no relief. So when something new comes along, like PEMF therapy, they hesitate. Not because they don't *want* it to work but because they're afraid it won't. They're worried it's just another failure waiting to happen. Another waste of time, money, and hope.

A lot of people think PEMF therapy is snake oil, voodoo, or junk science, especially because most people first hear about it online, and there's a lot of garbage out there. But the science is real, and the results are measurable. When you actually examine the studies, the history, the technology, and the outcomes, you'll see it's not magic. It's quantifiable energy applied to the body to help the body do what it's already designed to do: heal itself.

I hear it all the time: "I've tried everything, Mark. Will this really work?"

And my answer is always the same: "Maybe. Nothing is 100%. But maybe this is the thing that will change everything for you."

In the medical world, we often discuss "evidence-based" approaches and "double-blind" studies, but let's not forget that, in 2025, most pain is still measured using a smiley face chart—the AVS scale. You've seen it. Zero is a happy face. Ten is a guy in agony. The gold standard for assessing pain still boils down to:

"How bad is it today?"

"How bad is it now?"

That's subjective.

However, there are also *objective* tools. You can track your progress with wearables like a Fitbit, an Apple Watch, or an Oura Ring. These measure things like heart rate variability and stress. You can test blood markers like cytokines or even use expensive diagnostics to track changes in PTSD indicators at the cellular level. You can *see* and *measure* PTSD in the cell. We're currently sourcing our own wearable tech to help customers track objective results while using PEMF, as seeing is believing.

And I'll be the first to admit—I still don't believe it 100% of the time. And I'm a rocket scientist who has been studying this stuff for over 27 years. But the results keep showing up. Over and over again. In the numbers. In the stories. In the people who get their life back.

I even wrote an article for the Facebook haters called *Liar, Liar, Pants on Fire*. Because people online love to scream "Scam!" without doing an ounce of their own research. But here's a quote I live by:

> *"Any sufficiently advanced technology is indistinguishable from magic."*
> **—Arthur C. Clarke**

Do you know what else was once considered a scam? DNA sequencing. CRISPR. Antibiotics. Satellite communication. MRIs. At one point in time, each of those world-changing technologies was laughed at, mocked, dismissed, or deemed "impossible." But now? We use them every day without a second thought. The MRI is one of the most incredible machines ever invented. It's literal magic in a metal tube. And yet, nobody questions it now.

So when people look at PEMF and say, "That can't possibly work," I just nod. Because that's exactly what they said about every breakthrough that came before it.

Another reason people are suspicious about energy therapy is because *I'm* the one talking about it. My own sister asked me, "How can you even be doing this if you're not a doctor?" However, let me explain why that might be a good thing.

Doctors treat people with the tools they've been handed, most of which come straight from pharmaceutical reps. They're trained to use what's already accepted by the system. The problem is the system moves at the speed of sludge. On average, it takes 15 years for a new medical technology to go mainstream. And while they're slow to adopt the new, they're even slower to let go of the old.

As a rocket scientist, I don't have to wait for anyone's permission to explore what works. I get to chase what's effective, even if it's unconventional, especially if it's unconventional.

Many doctors are hesitant to use PEMF technology simply because it's under $1,000. If it doesn't cost tens of thousands or come with a substantial recurring income, then most medical professionals aren't interested. There are 15 middlemen in the healthcare food chain, from insurance to hospitals to manufacturers, and if each one doesn't get their cut, the product gets buried.

If you feel like the system is working against your health, you're not imagining it. When I tell people the FDA is trying to shut me down, their response is almost always the same:

"Yeah, that doesn't surprise me at all."

The FDA is not out here protecting your wellness. The drug companies don't want to make you better. They want to keep you sick, just functional enough to keep needing their products. Most doctors don't want to learn anything new. I call it the AMA Wall—the invisible barrier of the American Medical Association that stops your doctor from even considering something outside of what they're told.

This actually happened: I walked into my doctor's office with a summary I'd written—pages of research on cholesterol and blood pressure, things I've studied obsessively. I handed it to her and said, "Would you read this?"

She literally turned her face away and said, "I don't want to see that. I don't care what it says. I'm only going to do what the American Medical Association tells me."

She didn't want to know more. She didn't want to question. She just wanted to stay in line. That's what we're dealing with.

Doctors aren't bad people. But they are trapped in a system that *rewards compliance* and *punishes curiosity,* which is built on what's called "standard of practice," and here's where it gets laughable. The concept of "standard of care" in medicine dates back to a lawsuit involving coal barges in the early 1900s. A storm hit, barges sank, and everyone sued everyone. The court ruled that since radios existed at the time, a responsible barge operator should have had one to hear the weather reports. That became the legal foundation for what's now used in medical lawsuits: if you didn't follow the *standard of practice*, you're liable. So, doctors hide behind the AMA and follow the rules. Even if something better exists, they won't touch it unless the system says it's okay. Because if something goes wrong, they want to be able to say, "I did what the standard told me to do."

Even if that standard is 20 years outdated and no longer works.

If you've been wondering why PEMF isn't everywhere, why your doctor hasn't recommended it, or why insurance won't cover it—this is why.

Because your wellness doesn't serve their business model.

Because healing you would break the system.

Because there's too much money in keeping you coming back.

That's why something affordable, accessible, and *effective* like PEMF makes people uncomfortable. It works without feeding the system. And trust me, when you start diving into how the insurance companies artificially jack up prices, you'll feel sick. There are entire podcasts and exposés dedicated to showing just how corrupt that world really is.

Be skeptical. I encourage it. But don't stop there. Do your homework. Because if you can look past the noise, beyond the fear, and outside the system that's profiting from your pain, you might just find something that works.

I'm sure you have some of the same questions everyone else does:

"Does it really work?"

You've tried things that didn't work, things that made it worse, or things that cost a fortune and gave you nothing in return. So, when someone tells you that a small, pocket-sized device can help you finally get some relief, your first question is, of course, *really?*

"How can something so small and simple be effective?"

It doesn't plug into the wall. It doesn't make any noise. It doesn't buzz, beep, or light up like a Christmas tree. It simply *works* by communicating with your body in its own language—energy. And while that might sound strange at first, the most powerful technologies in the world often start out looking like magic.

"Is it safe?"

Not only is PEMF therapy non-invasive and drug-free, but it's also one of the gentlest, most natural methods of supporting your body's healing process. You don't have to worry about harmful side effects, withdrawals, or mixing it with other treatments. It won't shock your system. It will restore balance.

In the chapters ahead, we'll walk through how this technology works, why it's been hidden from you, and how people just like you are using it to reclaim their lives and rediscover joy.

No, I'm not a doctor. I don't have a white coat, and I'm not going to rattle off a bunch of Latin terminology to impress you. I'm an engineer. I was a chief engineer on the Space Shuttle—and to my knowledge, I was the youngest one ever at just 31 years old.

But my journey into energy therapy didn't start in a lab. It started with my dog. She had bad arthritis. And no vet, no drug, no surgery could help her. The *only* thing that could work was this strange, advanced technology—PEMF. And 27 years ago, that technology wasn't something you could pick up on Amazon. You had to drive two states away to find a clinical setup that had one. It was expensive, rare, and *inaccessible*. But it worked. And once I saw what it could do, not just for my dog, but for people struggling with PTSD, I couldn't unsee it. And frankly, I got mad. Because healing shouldn't be locked behind money or gatekeepers. You shouldn't have to be rich or desperate to find something that helps you feel human again.

So, I approached this like an engineer would:

How can I make this smaller?
How can I make it affordable?
How do I get this into the hands of real people who need it most?

That's been my mission ever since. Not to play doctor. But to solve the problem that no one else seemed interested in solving. This book is part of that mission.

I want you to wake up smiling, not screaming. I want you to sleep through the night for the first time in a long time so you can feel like yourself again and do things you haven't done in twenty years—go for a walk, laugh at a joke, and enjoy time with people you love. You should be in control of your health, your day, and your emotions.

One of the best measures of success is the feedback I hear all the time when your friends and family start saying:

"You're different."

"You're back."

Because when you're in pain, especially long-term emotional or physical pain, you *can't* see yourself clearly. You can't read the label from inside the bottle. Sometimes, it takes someone else to tell you that you're finally showing up in the world differently. People forget how bad they felt. I've seen it happen over and over. I'll be on a Zoom call with someone who says, "Eh, I don't know if it helped that much..."

And I'll pull out their numbers— "You went from a 72 to a 12 on the PTSD scale in 30 days."

They look at the screen, and they cry. Because they forgot. That's how powerful and subtle real healing can be. My theory is it's like childbirth. If women remembered *exactly* how painful it was, no one would ever have a second kid. However, they do because the brain *releases* that pain once the body is whole again. The same thing happens here.

I wrote this book because I want you to know there *is* another way. There is hope. And it doesn't require a prescription, a pile of cash, or blind faith in a broken system. Also—I'm 64, so I don't have forever to get my message out. This is one more way for me to make noise, to turn up the volume on a message that *everyone* needs to hear. And yeah, I have dreams of going on *Shark Tank*, standing in front of Mark Cuban, and saying, "I'm looking for $0 for 10% of my company—and you, Mark, are already out because you always torpedo any new health technology."

Not for the deal. For the *platform*. Because if people like him won't listen, maybe the rest of the world will.

My words are grounded in 27 years of real-world learning, engineering, and witnessing people's lives transform. If you've been struggling with anxiety, emotional pain, or chronic frustration and nothing has worked, this book is for you. You don't have to believe me yet. Just stay curious.

Let's get started.

- Mark L. Fox

PART ONE
Rethink Anxiety

CHAPTER ONE

The Anxiety Puzzle You've Been Trying to Solve

Anxiety is the most common ailment in people and pets around the world. And honestly, I find that strange. You'd think we'd understand it better by now. If it's the number one issue people are facing, why aren't we discussing *why* it happens more?

I've always been curious. Not necessarily a tinkerer like some engineers, but someone who constantly asks *why*. And when it comes to anxiety, I still don't have the perfect answer. But I can't help wondering. Why do people get more fearful as they get older? Is it genetic? Is it just part of aging? That doesn't quite make sense to me.

And what about animals? Why was my dog so afraid of being left behind when we'd go flying and camping? We'd take the

Cessna 182 and go plane camping, and she was always nervous. We'd get to the end of a trail, turn back, and she'd take off in a full sprint back to the plane—like we were going to leave her. And we never had.

At its core, anxiety might come down to that: fear of the unknown. And if that's true, then it may help explain many things, such as why religion persists. People often struggle to explain how we arrived here, what the universe is, and why we exist. So, we create frameworks to make sense of it. Maybe anxiety comes from that same place, trying to make sense of things we don't fully understand.

Speaking personally, I've had a lot of anxiety around health, especially around blood pressure. In college, I was about to graduate and join the Army. To get cleared, you had to get your blood pressure taken twice a day for two weeks. Mine was perfectly normal the whole time until the very last day.

That day, a new nurse walked in. Very attractive. She took my arm, slid my hand under her armpit—so my hand was on her breast—and then took my blood pressure. It spiked to something like 200 over 100. She looked surprised. "You had great numbers before—what happened?" I said, "Maybe it's the person taking it." She got offended, threw the clipboard down, and stormed out.

Then they sent in the older, grumpy nurse, and my blood pressure returned to normal. But it didn't matter. I had now officially violated some Army protocol. The next thing I know, I'm being told I might lose my commission. I had no apartment, no place to live, and the Army might not take me. That's when I realized that anxiety doesn't always have a clear cause. Sometimes, it's just there, and sometimes it spirals into something bigger because of the *reaction* to it.

I'm a pilot. Pilots are required to undergo regular health checks, including blood pressure screenings. If it's too high, you risk losing your license. Think about the commercial pilots out there—guys making $200,000 a year—sitting there checking their blood pressure over and over before an appointment to make sure they pass. That kind of stress *creates* high blood pressure.

And then you've got doctors who don't help the situation. One time, a doctor told me my pressure was high and that I should double my medication. I didn't want to, but he insisted. So I did. And it nearly killed me. My blood pressure dropped so low I couldn't even get off the couch to call 911.

I went back to him later and said, "You almost killed me."

His response? "It's not an exact science, Mark. It's called *practicing* medicine for a reason."

And speaking of the doctor, you know what nobody ever asks you at the doctor's office?

"What would you like to get out of this relationship?"

Not one nurse or doctor I've ever met starts a session with that question. And it's a shame because that alone would lower a lot of people's anxiety, including mine.

Instead, you're herded into a freezing cold room, rushed in and sat down, and within seconds—*boom*—they slap the cuff on and take your blood pressure. No waiting the recommended 15 minutes. No calm. Just the cattle system in full force.

And then, if your numbers are high, which of course they are in that environment, they start making the "nurse face." You know the one. Eyebrows raised, concerned noises, maybe a gasp or two. And just like that, you feel ten times worse. It's never helpful when they say, "Just go to your happy place." That doesn't work for me. It draws attention to the anxiety. It's like saying, "Don't think about the elephant in the room." Now you're absolutely thinking about the elephant.

If I could have an honest conversation where someone asked me what I needed, what would help, or which parts of the process stress me out, I know my anxiety would go down.

This chapter is important because anxiety isn't a clear-cut condition. Sometimes there's a reason, sometimes there's not, and most of the time, it's some confusing blend of both. But what's *not* the answer, at least not the full answer, is just throwing drugs at it and hoping for the best.

We can do better. We need to understand it better. And that starts with asking questions, being curious, and not accepting surface-level solutions to something that touches so many lives every single day.

Many people think anxiety is purely mental. Or they say it's chemical. But they're missing a big piece of the puzzle. We're not just physical and chemical beings—we're *electrical*, too. Your body operates on all three levels: physical, chemical, and electrical. And when we ignore that third piece, we're throwing the whole system out of balance.

You've probably heard of Dale Carnegie and Rockefeller. Well, Rockefeller figured out how to make drugs from oil, and since he owned all the oil in the country, guess what happened? We ended up with a medical system focused almost entirely on drugs and surgery. That was great for him. It's not so great for the rest of us. We abandoned the electrical side of our biology. We stopped talking about it and treating it. And that's just plain stupid. Because if your body is physical, electrical, and chemical, and we're only paying attention to two out of the three, we're not getting the whole picture, not for people, not for pets, not for anybody. And that's precisely why we're so far behind in the U.S. when it comes to things like electrical stimulation. We've ignored it for too long, and we're paying the price.

■ *If You Can't Burn It, It Isn't Real?*

Let me give you a different angle on how the medical system handles anxiety and why so many people get told, "It's all in your head."

I was at the Wizard Academy over a decade ago. Kerry Mullis was there, the guy who won the Nobel Prize for inventing PCR, the polymerase chain reaction. He's a big deal in the world of chemistry. Brilliant guy. Total materialist. His thinking was very much, *"If you can't see it, touch it, smell it, or burn it—it isn't real."*

So there we were, maybe a hundred, hundred-fifty people in the room, and Roy Williams was on stage talking about marketing. I've heard Roy say it a hundred times: *"Where the heart goes, the mind will follow."* In other words, people make decisions emotionally and then gather facts to support their existing feelings.

Roy challenges Kerry right there. He says, "Kerry, come up here." Then he asks him this simple question:

"Does your mother love you?"

Kerry's like, "What?"

Roy says again, "Does your mother love you?"

Kerry finally answers, "Yes."

And then Roy says, "Prove it. Smell it. Taste it. Burn it."

And Kerry just... breaks. Right there, on stage. He starts to cry. And Roy looks at the audience and says, "Exactly."

That moment stuck with me. Because it showed how even the most intelligent minds can fall into the trap of thinking that if something is not measurable, it's not real. And the entire medical system has bought into that mindset. You go in for your annual physical. You get 10 minutes if you're lucky with the doctor. And most of what they tell you is based on the results of your blood test. Because that's the measurable stuff they can quantify. If it's not showing up in those numbers, then you're fine.

So what happens when someone comes in with anxiety, trauma, or unresolved nervous system overload?

They tell you it's all in your head.

Not because they're mean. Not because they don't care. But because the system they operate in only validates what can be tasted, touched, smelled, or burned. And since there's no blood test for anxiety, they don't know what to do with it. They don't have the tools. They don't have the time. And they sure don't have the incentive.

Here's something else to question. If you ever get a blood test and one of your numbers is outside the "normal" range, ask your doctor where that range comes from.

Chances are they can't tell you.

That's because companies like Quest Diagnostics and the drug manufacturers *set the ranges*. And they can and do change them. I remember when "normal" blood pressure was 120 over 80. Then, one day, it quietly became 115 over 75. No major studies announced it; it just changed.

So I asked the question: *Why?* Where's the data proving that 115 over 75 is better for people, especially as they age? I couldn't find it.

I did find that these companies move the goalposts because it helps sell more drugs. You bring the range down, and suddenly, more people are "outside" the norm, and now they qualify for a prescription. That's not healthcare. That's marketing.

Now, when a doctor tells me my blood pressure is high, I ask, "What do you think it should be for someone who's 64 years old?"

They usually say, "120 over 80."

I tell them, "Actually, it should be 140 over 90."

And I've got the data to back that up—a meta-analysis with 450,000 participants. The most extensive study of its kind. It removed doctor bias completely. The conclusion? For people over 60, trying to drive blood pressure down to 120 over 80 actually *increases* risk. Your body needs a bit more pressure to function well with age.

One doctor even told me, "Don't show me that study—I'm not going to look at it."

That's where we are.

So yes—the system reinforces the idea that anxiety is "just in your head" because it's been conditioned only to respect what can be measured on a lab sheet. But the human body is far more than numbers on a printout. It's electric. It's emotional. It's dynamic. And sometimes, it's carrying things that no blood test could ever detect, which is what we will discuss next.

■ *Your Body Might Be Screaming—You're Just Not Hearing It That Way*

Anxiety doesn't always show up as anxious thoughts. Sometimes, it shows up as stomach issues, neck pain, back pain, or constipation. I mean, pick a symptom, and there's a decent chance it could be rooted in nervous system dysregulation.

I have a friend who has been suffering from severe stomach pain and cramps for years. They thought he had stomach cancer. They ran every test and couldn't figure it out. They were about to cut his stomach out and do all kinds of wild surgeries, even thinking it might be testicular cancer at one point. He said it felt like someone hit him in the nuts with a baseball bat.

Then a psychologist finally unraveled the truth: he had been raped as a kid by a priest and had completely blocked it out. Once that trauma surfaced and he started working through it, *all* the physical pain started going away.

That's what anxiety and trauma can do. It hides. It waits. And if you're not tuned into it—or if your doctors are only looking at lab results and not listening to your life story—you'll miss the real cause.

I made up a word (because doctors do it all the time): **Diabiological Syndrome**. DIA as in *Depression, Insomnia, Anxiety*. And the thing is, those three always run together. You can't sleep because you're anxious. You're depressed because you can't sleep. You're anxious because you're depressed. Round and round it goes.

But this isn't just a theory. A friend of mine is writing a book on this exact topic, and he told me about a patient who was on four medications, had a blood sugar of 350, and couldn't get it down. Then, her daughter moved out of the house, and her blood sugar dropped to 100, and she's off all meds and feeling fantastic.

Stress can jack your system up to the point where you're getting diagnosed with chronic diseases and prescribed drugs when what you really need is healing from the inside out.

Let's revisit blood pressure for a moment, as this one drives me crazy. I've dealt with it personally for decades. And here's what I finally heard—*from one doctor ever*—that stuck with me:

"High blood pressure by itself isn't dangerous. It's a symptom telling you something else is going on."

That blew my mind. And it made sense. Sometimes, mine is high because I'm anxious about it being high, and I know they're about to take it. And that fear feeds itself. At other times, it might be signaling something else in the body.

But here's where things really went off the rails.

There was a drug that was once widely used in hospitals. When people came in having a stroke, doctors assumed the high blood pressure was causing the stroke. So they gave them this drug to bring it down.

What they didn't realize was that the blood pressure *wasn't* the problem—it was the body's way of compensating for the issue. The brain wasn't getting enough blood, so the body cranked up the pressure to try to deliver more. The drug stopped that, the pressure dropped, and people died. Lots and lots of them. The exact number will never be known. Silently.

Eventually, that drug disappeared from hospitals. No explanation. Just gone. Because someone finally realized that your body is trying to help you. You just aren't listening.

■ *The Vagus Nerve: Your Body's Superhighway*

We're learning so much more now about the vagus nerve, and honestly, it's fascinating. It's one of the only nerves in your body that goes both ways—your brain talks to your organs, *and* your organs talk back to your brain. It's the central highway connecting it all.

So if your vagus nerve is out of tune—if your body's in a constant fight-or-flight state—you'll feel it everywhere, especially in your digestion. And what we're seeing now in the studies we're doing is that once people tone the vagus nerve, those digestive issues begin to resolve. You calm the nerve; you calm the body.

You're Not Broken. You're Just Out of Power.

Here's a mindset shift I want you to try.

What if your body isn't broken?

What if it's just *out of power*?

That's one of the key messages I aim to convey when teaching creative thinking. And one of my favorite ways to illustrate this is with a little help from Pixar Animation Studios.

Think about what Pixar does with storytelling. They take something ordinary, such as a rat, a car, or a toy, and shift the viewpoint. Suddenly, you're seeing the world through the rat's eyes as it whips up a gourmet meal or the car's as it crosses the finish line. That shift brings the story to life. You start to understand things in a completely different way simply because of a new perspective.

So, let's do the same with your body. Try seeing your symptoms not as flaws but as messages. Instead of thinking, *"I'm broken,"* try thinking, *"My system is out of tune."*

Because it's true, your body isn't malfunctioning; it's trying to get your attention.

■ Quiet Again

I had a client named Ava who had always lived with anxiety. Even as a kid, her thoughts ran like a motor with no off switch. Over time, she learned how to mask it. She got good at functioning during school, work, or social events, but underneath, there was always that hum of unease she couldn't quite turn down.

She'd been on medication since her teens. It took the edge off, but it also muted everything else. She wasn't spiraling, but she wasn't really living either. It was strictly survival.

Then, in her 30s, Ava started having episodes that felt like heart attacks with chest tightness, racing pulse, and shallow breaths. She went through the whole medical gauntlet of EKGs, stress tests, and cardiologists. Everything came back normal. Her heart was fine, which left her even more confused. If her heart was healthy, why did it feel like it was ready to explode?

That's when someone pointed her in our direction. She came across our Anxiety protocol and started using the VIBE every day. Nothing dramatic happened at first. But by the end of the first week, she noticed something that stopped her in her tracks.

She had gone the whole morning without clenching her jaw.

That might not sound like much, but to her, it was like discovering silence after a lifetime of noise. She wasn't waking up already braced for the day. Conversations didn't drain her. Her mind felt steadier. For the first time in years—maybe ever—she wasn't stuck in fight-or-flight.

With her doctor's help, Ava started reducing her medication. Bit by bit, she cut it by more than half. And instead of feeling more anxious without it, she felt more like herself. She described it as coming back online, steady, clear, and calm. Her heart was never the problem. It was her nervous system screaming for help. And once she learned how to listen and recharge, it finally got quiet again.

■ *There Is Hope*

I didn't believe in PEMF at first. Not even a little. As a rocket scientist, it just sounded like a bunch of frequency voodoo. But what changed everything for me was PTSD.

I started seeing what PEMF could do for people dealing with severe trauma. Real stories. Real results. And that's what made me mad. Here was something that worked, yet hardly anyone had access to it. So, I dug deeper. I looked at the data. I started connecting the dots between PTSD, anxiety, the vagus nerve, and nervous system balance. And I thought, *'Why isn't this being used more widely?'*

So, we built protocols. Four of them: Anxiety, Relax & Balance, Vagus Nerve, and PTSD. All are designed to target the same issue—nervous system overload—from different angles, frequencies, and pathways to calm. We just kicked off our own clinical trial. And you know what I'm telling participants? *Alternate the protocols. See what works best for your system.*

Anxiety doesn't wear the same face for everyone. And sometimes, even the thing that's *supposed* to help you, like trying something new, can trigger fear. That's okay. It's all part of learning how to listen to your body and give it what it really needs.

At first, I thought PEMF might only be helpful for military vets dealing with PTSD. But the more we have worked, the more I have realized that there are just as many, if not more, civilian women walking around with deep, invisible wounds. Anxiety from trauma, abuse, toxic relationships, miscarriages, motherhood. Anxiety from growing up in a world that demands too much and gives too little.

And teenage girls? I see it all the time here at Cocoa Beach. They're out there on the sand, snapping photo after photo, posting to social media, waiting for the likes and the comments. And I can't help but wonder, what happens when someone says something cruel? What does that *do* to a young nervous system that's already hanging on by a thread?

We are all aware of the impact that phones and social media are having on the brain. And we all know anxiety is not some fringe issue. It's *everywhere*.

But so is hope.

If you're reading this and thinking, *This sounds like me*—I want you to hear me loud and clear:

There's hope.

That's it. That's what I want you to know first and foremost. There's hope for a better tomorrow. You are not alone. You are not broken. You are not weak. You're just a human being in an overstimulated world, doing your best to survive something that was never meant to be handled alone.

And don't let the **bozone** get in your way.

That's one of my favorite old words from Rich Hall back in the day—"bozone," like a mix between bozo and ozone. It's an invisible gas that blocks new ideas from getting in. We all carry a little bozone around with us sometimes. It's that voice that says, *No way in hell this is going to work.*

But if you can drop the bozone for a minute and keep your mind open, you might find something that changes everything. Look at the data. Try what resonates. Trust what your body tells you because your body *isn't* the enemy. It's your partner. And it's been trying to tell you something all along. You just have to start listening.

KEY TAKEAWAYS

- Anxiety isn't just in your head—it's often your nervous system trying to send a message, and ignoring that message can lead to even bigger issues.

- Our current medical system overlooks the electrical side of human biology, focusing only on what can be measured or medicated, which leaves many people misunderstood and mistreated.

- Symptoms like high blood pressure, stomach pain, or insomnia may actually be signs of nervous system overload, not isolated health issues.

- Tools like PEMF and protocols focused on the vagus nerve can help calm the body's internal chaos by restoring balance to the system rather than just muting symptoms.

- You're not broken; you're out of power. But there's hope, and real solutions exist if you're willing to stay curious, listen to your body, and keep an open mind.

CHAPTER TWO

When the Modern World Throws Chaos Your Way

Stress isn't occasional anymore. It's ambient. Constant. It's everywhere, all the time. And if you feel like you're not handling life as well as you "should," you're not broken. You're just bombarded. Our brains were never meant for this. We weren't designed to deal with 46,000 emails, the dopamine loop of social media likes, online haters, and "always-on" digital everything. We were built for survival—gathering food, watching for danger, and resting in between. So it's no wonder we're anxious. It's the world we're living in. And the truth is, you can't really escape it. Not entirely. But you *can* understand it. You *can* learn how to handle it differently.

I'll give you an example. We've been working on a device called the Kario smartwatch. It's like a Fitbit but built with our own tech, tuned to what really matters for people who deal with stress, anxiety, and nervous system overload. One of its functions is to monitor blood pressure in real time.

I've had my own lifelong freak-out around blood pressure. Just the thought of it could get me worked up. Even going in for a basic physical, I'd start spinning in my head. Am I going to get into a fight with the doctor? Are they going to freak out? Am I going to freak out?

When we started testing the Kario watch, I was actually *afraid* to turn on the blood pressure feature. Because of my anxiety, I didn't want to see what it would say. But then, plot twist—it had already been on. The watch had been taking my blood pressure for two weeks, and I didn't even know it.

And it was normal. No danger. It was only ever bad when I'd get myself all worked up at the doctor's office. That right there was a 40-year weight off my shoulders. I realized the *anxiety* was real, but the *cause* wasn't. Or at least, it wasn't justified. Data has the power to prove to your nervous system that everything is okay.

That's one of the reasons we're developing the Kario watch. Because while PEMF therapy is an incredible tool for calming the system, the other half of the equation is feedback. You need a way to objectively *measure* what's changing. Your brain is looking for certainty, and data can help provide it.

So this topic is personal for me. And if you're feeling overwhelmed by life, or wired all the time, or like your body won't chill out, you're not alone. You're just living in the chaos of the modern world.

■ *Micro-Threats Are Everywhere*

Fight or flight isn't just triggered by the big, obvious stressors. It's the little stuff that I refer to as "micro-threats." Every time your phone buzzes with a notification—text, email, Slack ping, social media alert—your nervous system receives a little jolt. Your biology reads that alert as a possible threat. Multiply that by 10,000 a day, and no wonder we can't relax.

And don't get me started on the news. I'll flip on the national news maybe once every two weeks, and within 20 seconds, I'm pissed off and turning it off again. It's always something horrific—another shooting, another bombing, another doomsday scenario. Fear is the currency of media now.

It's the same with drug commercials. They start with "Do you feel anxious?" and end with "Ask your doctor about our magic pill... but side effects include death, by the way." I mean, come on.

Then there's social media. That's a whole other kind of stress. Every "like," every comment, every share becomes a scorecard. Am I good enough? Do people care? Why did their post do better than mine? Why do they seem to have it all together while I don't? It's a nonstop loop of comparison, which messes with your head in ways you don't always see right away.

The sneaky part is most of the triggers I'm referring to are invisible. They don't seem like threats. They're just "normal" parts of your day. But they're baked into your routine so deeply that your nervous system never gets a break.

Blue light from screens that keeps you up at night. Sitting too long and never getting real movement. The idea is that if you're not constantly multitasking, you're lazy. We've created this unrelenting productivity culture where if you're not doing a thousand things, you feel like you're falling behind.

Think back to the old days when people's biggest worry was, "Did I plant enough crops before winter?" They didn't have to deal with 50 app notifications and breaking news about the latest disaster every hour. Their lives weren't easier, but they were *simpler*. Simplicity lets your nervous system reset.

■ *Perception vs. Reality*

The nervous system reacts to *perceived* danger. And that's where everything gets scrambled. When I worked on the space shuttle, I was often asked: "Is it safe to launch?" There's no simple answer to that. You can't list 22,000 known defects that were all reviewed, dispositioned, and engineered to be *acceptable*. That would take too long. So we just had to say yes or no.

But I started wondering—what does "safe" even mean?

I looked it up. The dictionary says, *free from risk or harm*. But that's not accurate. You can choke on food, crash your car, or get taken out by a falling tree branch on a calm day. There's risk in *everything*. So, I came up with my own definition. Safety is when the *perceived* benefits outweigh the *perceived* risks.

That's how we make almost every decision in life. We get up, we go to work, and we make plans—all based on how our brain is weighing benefits and risks at that moment. The problem is those are just *perceptions*. Yours. Mine. And they can be totally different. That's why negotiating with someone or even having a conversation can go sideways—because their perceived pros and cons don't match yours at all. And none of it's "real." It's just interpretation.

Think about it. Your brain processes a perceived threat in thousandths of a millisecond. You slam on the brakes because something darted across the road. You didn't have time to think it through. That's your nervous system doing its job.

But what happens when that same system gets triggered by modern life—by stuff like deadlines, notifications, or traffic? It *still* reacts, just like it would to a tiger. That's the mismatch. That's where the chaos comes in. You've got an old system doing what it was designed to do in a world that has moved at an exponential pace. And it hasn't caught up.

■ *When Survival Mode Becomes Your New Normal*

When your nervous system is activated by stress over and over, it doesn't go back to neutral. It starts to *stay* in survival mode. That "always on" setting becomes the new baseline. The real problem is it stops feeling weird. The emergency signal—tight chest, shallow breathing, racing thoughts—starts to feel *normal*. Your body forgets what calm feels like.

Even for me, it's tough sometimes. I've had moments where I'm sitting on a beach, just watching the waves, and I can't relax. Calm feels *foreign* as if I should be doing something, solving something, and working on the next thing. The world has wired us to stay revved up, and eventually, that becomes hard to undo.

It's like you're driving a car with one foot on the gas and one foot on the brake. You're not in cruise control. You're in constant anticipation of something going wrong. Unless you take deliberate action to break that cycle—such as using PEMF, meditation, or any other method that gives your system a reset—it will just continue. Meditation has made its way into boardrooms and businesses now because people are finally realizing they need 40 minutes *not* to be on.

So, what does this "always on" state look like in your body? You can't sleep. You've got gut issues. You're bloated or nauseous. You grind your teeth at night. Your muscles are tense, your blood pressure's up, and your immune system starts tanking.

One of the biggest things we're seeing more of is problems with the *vagus nerve,* the command center for rest and repair in your body. And if it's not toned—meaning, if it's not functioning properly—your body literally can't heal. It doesn't matter if it's the flu, a stomach issue, or something way more serious. Without vagus nerve tone, the body is not receptive to healing at the cellular level.

I discussed this on a recent podcast. A doctor told me, "You can't heal from *anything* unless your vagus nerve is toned." It explains why so many people feel stuck in their recovery. The problem isn't just in your gut, or your sleep, or your immunity—it's in the *system* behind all those systems. And stress is the thing blocking the signal.

■ *Rest Is Recovery*

If you're scrolling Facebook in bed with the blue light blazing while your spouse is already asleep beside you, that's one of the worst things you can do for your sleep. You're basically telling your brain, "We're still in danger, don't calm down."

Instead, get rid of all electronic stimulation at least 30 minutes before bed—an hour if you can. Blue light, emails, social feeds... all of it. Shut it down. Overstimulation right before bed messes with your hormones, builds muscle tension, and fuels those racing thoughts where your mind spins about tomorrow's to-do list right when you're trying to fall asleep. We've all been there. And it's a cycle you can break—but you have to be intentional about it.

People tend to think, "I'm just tired; I need some rest." But real sleep isn't just about rest. It's about *recovery*. You *need* sleep so your cells can repair themselves. That's how your body moves from fight-or-flight into rest-and-digest.

One of the top indicators of vagus nerve health is heart rate variability. And what we're seeing in the data is that sleep plays a huge role in whether or not your vagus nerve is functioning the way it should.

Poor sleep and chronic stress often co-occur. You don't sleep well because you're stressed—and then, because you don't sleep, you get *more* stressed. It's a vicious cycle. And the problem is that many people have accepted it. They say things like, "I'm just a bad sleeper."

But maybe you're not. Perhaps it's not a flaw—it's a *pattern*. And maybe the way out isn't a sleep aid—it's dealing with the chronic nervous system stress you've been carrying for way too long. PEMF is one of the tools that can help interrupt that stress pattern. It helps shift your brainwaves out of the "amped up" beta state and move you toward theta, which is where deep, restorative sleep happens.

How I Finally Memorized the Brainwaves (And Maybe You Will Too)

If you've ever gotten confused about the brainwave states, you're not alone. I struggled with that for six months. I could never remember the order. So, I came up with this phrase that orders them from lowest to highest:

"Do the Atheists Believe in God?"

- **D** is Delta (deep sleep)
- **T** is Theta (relaxation/sleep)
- **A** is Alpha (calm/focused)
- **B** is Beta (active thinking)
- **G** is Gamma (intense cognition)

When your brain is stuck in high-beta because you're still processing input at 11 pm, your body doesn't get the chance to go down into theta and delta, where the real rest and repair happens. That's the shift we're trying to create. Put the phone down. Turn off the noise. Give your system a chance to power down. Your healing depends on it.

■ *Do Less—With Intention*

If you're looking for a couple of things you can do right now to push back against overstimulation, it's about doing *less* but doing it with intention.

I had this boss once, General Tom Honeywill—an old-school guy who kept a single daily 3x5 card in his pocket. One day, I noticed he only had *three* things written down. I told him, "They pay you way too much to only do three things a day." And he just said, "Let's talk at the end of the week and compare who actually finished more projects."

And guess what? He almost always did. Because I was trying to do 50 things and finishing none of them. Oversimplifying with intention is way more powerful than frantically chasing everything that feels urgent.

That's another thing I picked up from Roy Williams: *don't confuse what's merely urgent with what's important.* This little principle alone can change your entire relationship with stress.

Remember that apps and social platforms are *designed* to hijack your attention. The pings, buzzes, and notifications are all pulling you back into the system. Fight it. Turn off the notifications. I've done it, and it's tough at first, but the clarity that comes with silence is worth it.

Here's a simple habit: don't check your phone or computer for one hour *after* you wake up and one hour *before* bed. The morning window matters just as much as the bedtime impact. Let your brain *wake up* before you throw it into fight-or-flight.

■ *Become a Sailor*

You weren't designed to power through 24/7, to outrun stress, or to live in a loop of anxiety and tension. You were built to feel life, to experience it fully, to enjoy it. But to do that, you've got to reset your system. You've got to permit yourself to slow down, to get quiet, to *listen* to what your body is telling you.

And remember this—something we talk about all the time at the Wizard Academy: There are **drowners, floaters, surfers, and sailors.**

- **Drowners** sink. They're overwhelmed, going under, with no direction and no control.
- **Floaters** stay on the surface, but they drift wherever the current takes them—no real agency.
- **Surfers** ride the wave. That's better, but they still depend on the current. They go where the wave goes.
- **Sailors**—that's where you want to be. Sailors *navigate.* They've got a rudder, a sail, and a destination. Even when the wind is in their face, they find a way forward.

This book, this chapter—is encouraging you to become a sailor, not escaping the world, but learning to navigate it with calm, clarity, and control. No matter how loud things get, you *can* reclaim your peace.

KEY TAKEAWAYS

- You're not broken—you're overloaded by a modern world that constantly overstimulates your nervous system with micro-threats, notifications, and pressure to always be "on."

- Your body reacts to perceived threats in the same way it reacts to real ones, which means daily stressors like traffic, emails, and news can keep you stuck in a state of survival mode.

- Proper recovery starts with deliberate rest. PEMF therapy, improving vagus nerve tone, and reducing blue light and stimulation are key to resetting your system.

- Simplifying your days with intention, such as focusing on just a few priorities and avoiding constant phone checks, can have a greater impact than trying to accomplish multiple tasks simultaneously.

- You don't need to escape the chaos—you need to learn how to navigate it.

PART TWO

Ready To Reboot?

CHAPTER THREE

From Rocket Science to Nervous System Healing

If you've ever seen the movie *Apollo 13*, it's one of the most accurate depictions of a space disaster I've ever seen on screen. But more than the accuracy, there's a moment in that movie that I'll never forget—one of my favorite lines. The spacecraft has just suffered a catastrophic failure. Everyone in the NASA control center is screaming, panicking, and throwing ideas around. It's utter chaos.

Then Gene Kranz, the flight director, steps in and cuts through the noise. He drags on his cigarette, looks around, and says, *"Let's look at this from the standpoint of status. What do we got on the spacecraft that's still good?"*

He didn't focus on what was broken. He focused everyone on what was still working.

Just like that, he rebooted the entire room.

That moment is the perfect metaphor for what I'm trying to help people do with their nervous systems. We all need a reboot sometimes—not just our computers, phones, or TVs. Our nervous systems need it too. And if you're living with anxiety, chances are you're stuck in that mission control panic mode. Everything feels like it's breaking. Alarms are going off. But the real question is: *What do you still have that's good?*

This simple shift in perspective can change everything.

I teach a concept called business topology using TRIZ, a Russian theory of inventive problem-solving. The basic idea behind TRIZ is this: Every problem you're dealing with has already been solved somewhere—maybe not in your field, but in another one. And there are only about 40 different kinds of solutions. So creativity isn't necessarily about making something new. It's about seeing something from a different viewpoint and applying it to your situation.

It's the same with healing. You don't need to invent a whole new nervous system. You need to reboot it by looking at things in a way you never have before.

I've had my own reboots. I'm 64 now, but I didn't meet my birth mother until I was 48 years old. I found out she was homeless. That changed everything I thought I knew about myself and where I came from. For 48 years, I had this idea of who she might be, and then in an instant, my whole mental system rebooted. I had to update everything.

Shifting Perspective

When I talk about rebooting and shifting perspective, I sometimes liken my work to Pixar animations. As we discussed in Chapter One, Pixar introduces us to a rat that can cook (Ratatouille) or cars with emotions (Cars), showing us familiar things from entirely new angles. And that fresh viewpoint makes us feel something we didn't expect.

The same goes for upside-down maps. When you flip a world map and suddenly Australia's on top, your brain short-circuits for a second. It forces you to see the world differently. That's valuable.

And then there's the story of Joshua Bell. One of the greatest violinists in the world. He once played in a subway station, dressed like a regular guy. For hours, people rushed by without noticing him. He made seven bucks. Just the night before, he played in a sold-out concert hall where the cheapest ticket was $350. What changed? Not the music. Just the viewpoint. The context.

So why am I telling you all this? Because everything I've learned—from space systems to homeless shelters to subway stations—points to one thing: When your system feels overloaded, when anxiety takes over, the first step is shifting your perspective. Asking, *"What do I have that's still good?"*

■ *Mission Control Isn't in Houston— It's in Your Head*

When people ask me, "How did you go from rocket science to nervous system healing?" the answer is simple. The systems are the same. Rockets have sensors and telemetry systems, which include feedback loops that constantly send data to mission control. Your nervous system operates similarly. The brain, the vagus nerve, and your organs are all just sensors and feedback loops, sending information back and forth 24/7.

Think about autopilot. Rockets run on it. You don't steer one manually once it's up there—it flies itself, similar to your body. You're not manually controlling your heart rate or breathing every second. It's all automatic. Your nervous system is running the show, just like mission control runs a launch.

And just like in space, when something starts shaking, rattling, or going off course, you don't scrap the mission. You look at the data, shift the frequency, and find a better signal. Let's look at some examples.

Eyes, Rockets, and Resonance

I'll take you back to the STS-1 space shuttle mission. Astronauts John Young and Robert Crippen were doing their debrief, and someone asked, "Any issues up there?"

They hesitated, and then one of them said, "Yeah... my vision was blurred for the first couple of minutes." The other one nodded—same thing happened to him. They both couldn't see clearly until *exactly* the two-minute mark.

So, what happened at two minutes?

That's when the solid rocket boosters cut off.

The human eye has a natural resonant frequency of approximately 19 hertz. And we discovered the solid rocket boosters were vibrating at *exactly* 19 hertz. That vibration caused their eyeballs to shake, resulting in blurred vision. In aerospace, we were learning firsthand how frequency interacts with the human body.

The Woodpecker Problem

I credit woodpeckers with helping me realize the power of frequency. The external tank of the shuttle, the big orange one in the middle, has excellent insulation. And woodpeckers *love* it because it's easy to peck into, it's warm, and it's protected. In other words: perfect bird real estate.

Woodpeckers are clever little bastards. They would peck holes *in the ocean side* of the tank. That's the side opposite the launch tower, so we couldn't reach them to scare them off. And you can't just go blasting a shotgun near a rocket, right?

So we had to get creative. We started experimenting with *sound frequencies*. We tested various tones until we found the one they disliked the most. Our "Pecker Patrol" team (and, yes, we had t-shirts), was able to drive them off with the right frequency!

Rockets Have Emotions Too

This one may sound strange, but hear me out. The vagus nerve is like your emotional damping system. It helps regulate how intensely you react to the world. Rockets need damping systems, too.

Back on STS-1, the first time the shuttle went up, we had a serious issue. The shock wave from the solid rocket boosters came *roaring back* off the launch pad and slammed into the Orbiter. It knocked a bunch of the heat tiles loose, which protected the shuttle during reentry. That could've been catastrophic.

We built a giant water tank. One of my very first jobs was designing the plumbing to dump 300,000 gallons of water onto the launch pad in *20 seconds*. Next time you see a picture of a shuttle on the pad, look for that giant water tower beside it. In this case, we weren't just launching rockets. We were calming them down.

Everything I learned in aerospace made me realize how deeply connected frequency is to biology. Eyes vibrating at 19 hertz. Woodpeckers responding to sound. Rockets needing shock absorbers. It's all feedback, frequency, and function. And now, I use that same knowledge to help people reboot *their own* systems and reclaim calm from chaos.

■ *Prototype > Prescription*

The freedom to help people in this way comes from the difference between my world and the traditional medicine world. **Engineers operate on a prototype mindset**; doctors operate on a prescription mindset.

Doctors are trained to write scripts. Engineers are trained to build something quickly, test it, break it, and then rebuild it. That's what I live by. Whether I'm engineering, running Facebook ads, or developing new PEMF protocols, I ask myself: *How can I fail in two weeks?* Not because I want to fail, but because I want to learn fast.

I once severely messed up a project for an entrepreneur-investor I was working with. I braced myself for getting kicked off the team, until he said:

"If I get one out of ten from you, we win."

He was looking at it from a risk-reward lens. Ten ideas, one home run? That's a win. But a doctor *can't* be wrong nine times out of ten.

I Don't Need a Billing Code

I'm also not bound by insurance rules. I don't have to code conditions or justify treatments to a claims adjuster. I can look at something and say, "How do I fix this?" instead of "What will insurance cover?"

Doctors aren't allowed to think like that. Their system doesn't reward exploration. It rewards diagnosis and medication. That's why I wrote my second book, *Da Vinci and the 40 Answers*, which discusses creative problem-solving and how all of the world's problems can basically be solved with 40 core solutions—TRIZ again. That's how I think. That's how I *have to* think.

In the medical system, creativity doesn't get reimbursed. Most doctors are trained to *medicate first*. You come in with anxiety, you're probably walking out with a script for a benzo like Xanax or Ativan, or maybe an SSRI like Zoloft or Lexapro.

The reality is they've got ten minutes with you. Doctors don't get paid to be Dora the Explorer. They're paid to prescribe, to code, and to match symptoms with drugs. And that's a system problem. Not necessarily a doctor problem. Most of them genuinely want to help. But their hands are tied by protocols and billing codes. They don't have the time or permission to explore the root cause, dig into your nervous system, or teach you about the vagus nerve, arguably one of the most important systems in your body.

In fact, how many of you reading this have ever even had a doctor mention your vagus nerve? Or measure your heart rate variability?

I never have.

They'll check your blood pressure. Your temperature. Maybe run your labs. However, they won't discuss HRV or nervous system tone. And that's the crazy part: there's no blood test for anxiety. But there *are* reliable markers—like HRV—that correlate with vagus nerve function. And now, with new sensors and wearables (I'm wearing one right now), we can actually track that.

Still, it gets ignored.

■ *Why Frequency Medicine Is the Future*

The biggest difference between what we do and what traditional medicine offers is **that there are no side effects**. Watch any six o'clock news segment, and you'll see it—90% of every drug commercial is just a rapid-fire list of side effects: dry mouth, dizziness, suicidal thoughts, and the rest of the horror show.

People are waking up to that. And no, I don't mean "woke"— that word has been used to death. I mean *awake*. Aware. They're starting to realize they don't need to surrender their health to prescriptions and 10-minute doctor visits. They're tracking their vitals, running their own labs, and wearing sensors on their wrists. They're starting to ask better questions.

These days, most patients are more knowledgeable about their conditions than their doctors are, particularly in cases involving rare or complex situations. You get a serious diagnosis in the family, and suddenly you're reading every study, joining forums, and talking to experts. Meanwhile, your doctor's still using a standard flowchart from 2004.

People are realizing they've been misled. Sometimes on purpose. Sometimes, just because the "authorities" were uninformed. Doesn't matter which. The result is the same: we've been told the wrong things for decades.

I'm probably the only idiot you'll ever meet who actually reads the U.S. Dietary Guidelines every five years. They're maddening. First, they demonized eggs—eggs were evil. Then, after years of research proved they were actually good for you, did they admit they were wrong? No. They just skipped the chapter. Quietly moved on as if it had never happened.

Same with the fat-free craze. For 30 years, we were told fat was bad. So what happened? They pulled the fat and replaced it with sugar. Now we've got metabolic disease, obesity, and a population addicted to carbs. Don't even get me started on the salt myths. Salt's not the villain—it's misunderstood, just like so many other things.

Here's what it comes down to: **energy is the foundation of life, not chemistry.** People are beginning to get that. They're taking back control. Some may still wonder, "Isn't PEMF just more BS?"

That's the biggest misconception. People hear the term *"electromagnetic frequency"* and immediately associate it with EMF from Wi-Fi, 5G, or whatever else they've read in fear-mongering headlines.

PEMF devices *do* emit EMFs, but not all EMFs are bad.

The kinds we use are extremely low energy, and they're therapeutic. That's the key. They're designed to *help* the body regulate itself, not fry your insides. When someone asks me about this, I explain it like this:

Everyone's had a dental X-ray. That's EMF at the power of 10 to the 12th. Super intense. Now compare that to PEMF therapy—that's basically zero on the scale. Several trillion times weaker. It's not even in the same universe. But people hear "EMF" and assume "danger."

However, here's the reality. Frequency medicine is starting to show up in smart devices, wearables, and even your furniture. We're already inventing and testing technologies that embed healing frequencies into the things around you.

My dream—if I can ever find the right engineer—is to reverse the wireless charging coil in your phone. You know that coil that charges your device when you set it on a pad? A Qi Coil. If we could reverse the process and run an MP3 file "out" that same coil, we could turn *every cell phone* into a frequency therapy device.

Engineers keep telling me it's impossible. I just haven't found the wise one yet.

Another idea I've been chasing for years? Smart bulbs. Imagine saying, "Alexa, run depression protocol in the living room," and having the lights in your house pulse at the right frequency to help shift your emotional state. Now, you can't do that *yet*, because bulbs are built to power on with a slight delay, so they don't shock your eyes. But we're getting close. All I need to do is make a bridge around that delay.

And when it happens? You won't even know it's working. You'll just feel better. The room will feel better. The people in it will be calmer, clearer, and more balanced.

Because **your body is not a machine, it's a symphony.** And *you* are the conductor.

Frequency tools help you tune into the music that's already there—the music of joy, calm, clarity, who you are at your core.

We're not trying to eliminate stress altogether. Stress isn't the villain here. It's a necessary part of life. You *need* fight-or-flight when something's chasing you. But you also need calm, restoration, and balance. PEMF, vagus nerve stimulation, and all the technology we're referring to are helping your body return to its natural rhythm. The real healing happens when your nervous system knows how to dance again. And that's even deeper than rocket science.

KEY TAKEAWAYS

- Rebooting your nervous system starts with shifting perspective. Just like mission control, focus on what's still working, not just what's going wrong.

- Your body runs on feedback loops and resonance. Frequency plays a direct role in how we feel and function.

- Traditional medicine relies on prescriptions and protocols, while engineers build, test, and adapt, solving problems creatively rather than chemically.

- Frequency medicine isn't magic or a scam—it's low-energy, therapeutic, and already showing up in wearables, smart tech, and the environments around us.

- Your body is a symphony, and healing happens when you learn to tune it, not medicate it into silence.

CHAPTER FOUR

Your Body's Reset Button: PEMF Therapy Explained

L et me break this down as simply as I can: your cells are like tiny batteries. And when those batteries run low on juice—when their voltage drops—you get sick.

It really is that basic.

PEMF recharges your cells. Every cell in your body has a voltage, just like a car battery. That voltage is critical because it controls what gets in and out of your cells. With a strong charge, your cells can pull in the good stuff—nutrients, minerals, oxygen—and push out the bad stuff—waste, toxins, inflammation.

But if your cellular battery is low, the doors stay shut. You get sluggish; your metabolism tanks. Healing slows. You don't feel like yourself. And eventually, things break down.

The second thing PEMF does is boost your ATP production. That's adenosine triphosphate, a fancy word for the energy currency your cells run on. ATP is the fuel that powers everything your body does, from thinking clearly to digesting food to fighting off illness.

And here's the crazy part: PEMF can increase ATP by up to 500%, which is certainly not a little bump in energy. It's rocket fuel for your body's natural healing engine.

If you're trying to overcome anxiety, if your nervous system feels stuck in survival mode, you need your cells firing on all cylinders. Anxiety doesn't just live in your mind. It lives in your body. It's energy. It's chemistry. It's an electrical imbalance.

So what's the best way to fight an electrical problem? With an electrical therapy.

PEMF might sound like it's all about magnetism—and yeah, it is a pulsed magnetic field—but here's what most people don't realize: *alternating magnetic fields create small electrical currents in the body*. That's physics. That's Faraday's Law. And that current helps restore the body's natural rhythm.

The Body Doesn't Lie

I've told you the story of my dog, and I want to come back to it here, because it was my first real "aha" moment with PEMF. My dog had severe arthritis in her spine. I didn't know what else to do. Nothing was working. So I tried PEMF. And I saw it. You could *see* the change. She relaxed. She stopped yelping. Her movement improved.

No placebo effect. No power of positive thinking. Just real results on a dog who didn't know she was supposed to "feel better." That's when I realized something important: if it works on animals, for the most part, it's not a placebo. It's physics. You can't tell a horse to feel better. You can't coach a dog to relax.

But you *can* observe them.

With horses, you can look for signs such as licking and chewing, soft eyes, relaxed ears, and gentle nuzzling. With dogs, it's the direction of their tail wag, their body posture, and how alert or agitated they are. These are real, physical indicators that something inside is shifting. And these external cues, what I call "biomarkers," are often more honest than any pain scale a human might give you.

Even our so-called gold standard for measuring pain—the 0-to-10 analog visual scale—is still just subjective. But watching a dog calm down after PEMF is biology in action!

■ *How PEMF Interacts with the Vagus Nerve*

Let's talk about the vagus nerve for a minute. Because if you've been hearing more and more people mention it lately, you're not imagining things. The vagus nerve is getting attention because it has a huge impact on your health. It's one of the most powerful, misunderstood parts of your nervous system. And when you're in fight-or-flight mode—constantly anxious, reactive, burned out—it's often the vagus nerve that's out of tune.

One of the best ways to measure your vagus nerve tone is heart rate variability (HRV), which is the *variation* in time between your heartbeats. The higher your HRV, the more adaptable and resilient your body is.

High HRV = calm, balanced, responsive
Low HRV = stressed, reactive, fried

The chart below shows where your HRV should be depending on your age:

RMSSD: HOW DOES YOURS COMPARE?

Here's a guide to how RMSSD typically tracks across age groups and levels of recovery. These aren't rigid rules—just a snapshot of general trends.

Age Group	Excellent	Above Average	Average	Below Average	Poor
20-29 yrs	≥ 65 ms	55-64 ms	40-54 ms	30-39 ms	< 30 ms
30-39 yrs	≥ 60 ms	50-59 ms	35-49 ms	25-34 ms	< 25 ms
40-49 yrs	≥ 50 ms	40-49 ms	30-39 ms	20-29 ms	< 20 ms
50-59 yrs	≥ 45 ms	35-44 ms	25-34 ms	15-24 ms	< 15 ms
60+ yrs	≥ 40 ms	30-39 ms	20-29 ms	10-19 ms	< 10 ms

PEMF, especially our vagus nerve protocol, can help raise your HRV, creating more room between stressors and your reaction to them.

Tuning the Nerve... and the Brain

Here's where things get really interesting. When we discuss vagus nerve *stimulation*, most people picture some kind of zap or physical jolt. But PEMF works by using frequencies, the right kind of gentle, pulsed magnetic fields, that help tone the vagus nerve naturally.

Those same frequencies, particularly in the alpha and theta brain-wave ranges, not only tone the vagus nerve but also *entrain your brain* into a calmer state.

So it's a double win: your body gets calmer, and your brain learns what that calm feels like again. It's like putting the whole system back in harmony.

I like to think of PEMF as a gentle electrical coach for your vagus nerve. It doesn't yell. It doesn't force. It just *guides*. It helps your body say, "Hey, let's chill out. Let's slow this part down. Let's fire this up a bit."

It's biofeedback, in a sense, just one that your body already understands at an electrical level. It's like the system is listening and saying, "You're doing this too fast... too slow... let's bring it into balance."

And your body finally starts to exhale.

Atrial Fibrillation and the Vagus Nerve Surprise

I learned something wild in the last few weeks. We have customers using our vagus nerve protocol who are seeing their atrial fibrillation (AFib) drop dramatically. I'm talking about going from numbers like 50, 150, even 195 minutes a day of AFib… down to 2 minutes.

They're tracking it on their Apple Watches, and we're just now starting to piece it together. But it's working for some people in ways I never expected.

I just edited a video of a woman who had suffered for 25 years. Nothing worked. She tried everything. And now, with this protocol, she's sobbing on camera—just overwhelmed—because for the first time in decades, she found something that gave her real relief.

■ *"I Don't Feel Anything—*
So It Must Not Work"

People are used to therapy that feels like something. You take a pill, you feel a buzz. You use a TENS unit, and your muscles twitch. You go to a chiropractor, and you hear the crack.

The PEMF energy level is **a thousand times lower** than a TENS unit. So no, your muscles aren't going to contract. You won't feel it zapping you. It might not even make a sound, a light buzz at best.

That throws people off. They think, "Well, nothing's happening." But it *is*—it's just happening at the cellular level.

One of the most common reactions I hear from people in chronic pain is:

"Something's not right…"

But they say it with *relief.* It's this weird disorientation because they've lived with pain for so long that when it suddenly disappears, their brain doesn't know what to do with it. Their body feels… unfamiliar.

Then later they realize:

"Oh. My pain is gone."

Sometimes the relief hits so fast, it feels like being drunk or stoned. That's the endorphin dump. It's the runner's high, but without the running. I once had a woman in my office who'd been in a car wreck and had severe back pain for years. Within ten seconds of using PEMF, she said, "I need to sit down—I'm seeing double." The pain lifted so fast that her body couldn't keep up with the flood of feel-good chemicals it hadn't released in years.

So we tell people: *"Don't drive or operate machinery the first time you use this."*

Because you might get high on your own biology.

Why Some People *Do* Feel It

Now, here's something cool: a small percentage of people—like 1 to 3%—are energy sensitive. These folks feel the PEMF strongly. And for them, running the device at full power is *too much*.

Every time someone calls us and says, "It's broken!" nine times out of ten, they just turned the power down by accident. But the ones who say, "It's *too* strong..." those are the ones I always ask:

"Do you see colors or auras around people?"

And every single time, they are surprised: *"How the hell did you know that?"*

Because they do, they're tuned in differently. They walk into a room and can sense who's draining energy. And we've got enough data now to say—yep, if PEMF at a 10 setting is too much for you, you're probably one of those people.

For most people, you won't feel PEMF like a shock or a buzz. You'll just feel *better*. That might be calmer. Less anxious. More clear-headed. Less inflamed. Or, maybe—if you've been living in pain—you'll finally feel what it's like not to hurt. So don't dismiss it just because it's quiet. Sometimes the most powerful things work silently.

■ *The Secret Sauce: It's Easy*

With most interventions, people fall off. Every year, folks make resolutions—"I'm going to walk more, eat better, hit the gym"—and then life gets in the way. Even when your doctor tells you what to do, it's hard to fit it into your daily routine.

But with PEMF? You turn it on, drop it in your pocket, and forget it's even there.

Seriously. I can't tell you how many times I've reached for my phone in my pocket and realized it's not my phone, it's the VIBE—oh, I'm still running a protocol. I forgot I was even using it.

People continue to use it because it doesn't feel like "one more thing" to do. It doesn't interrupt their day. And that consistency gets results.

Now, don't get me wrong—other things work for anxiety. Tapping, breathwork, and medication. They all have their place. However, many of them come with baggage.

Meds? Side effects.

Tapping or breathing? You've got to remember to do them.

BEMER mats? They're powerful, but expensive. And unless you shell out $7,000 for one at home means you have to book appointments and go somewhere to use it.

That's where most people quit. Not because something didn't work, but because they couldn't stick with it. And if you stop showing up, the results will also stop showing up.

■ *Sleep Is the First Domino*

Speaking of results, one of the most common things I hear from people, sometimes even after their *first* session, is: *"I slept better than I have in years."*

Why is that?

Your brain spends most of the day in beta mode. That's your active, focused, maybe even slightly stressed-out state. But to sleep, you can't just slam on the brakes. You've got to *step down*.

The ideal path looks like this:
Gamma → Beta → Alpha → Theta → Delta

PEMF helps you walk that staircase naturally. When you use the Vagus Nerve Toning or Brainwave Alpha/Theta protocols, you're helping your brain move down from beta into alpha and theta. And *that* opens the path to delta, where real deep sleep occurs. Delta is your body's repair mode. It's where the magic of REM sleep, cellular healing, and emotional resetting takes place.

A Natural Boost in Melatonin and a Reduction in Everything That Keeps You Awake

PEMF has been shown to increase melatonin production, the hormone that tells your brain, "Hey, it's time to sleep." And it does that without a pill, without a prescription. You get there naturally.

It also reduces the things that keep you awake:

- **Pain and inflammation**: Whether it's restless legs, a throbbing knee, or a tight hip, when your body is lit up with discomfort, your mind can't settle. PEMF helps calm that down.
- **Monkey brain**: You know exactly what I'm talking about. You're lying there reliving every conversation from the day, rewriting your to-do list, and stressing about tomorrow. PEMF *quiets* that loop. It gives your mind permission to slow down.

And if that weren't enough, PEMF also increases blood flow, which supports detox, cellular repair, and overall brain function, critical stuff that happens while you sleep. It also lowers cortisol, the stress hormone that keeps your nervous system on high alert.

Christine G.

"After a decade of insomnia post-chemo, I now fall asleep in 5–10 minutes using Sleep and Brain Wave Delta. Prescription sleep aids didn't help, but this did. It's a miracle."

And it's not just people; it's animals, too. One of my favorite testimonials came from someone in the vibrational medicine world:

Sally H.

"Put on Brainwave Delta, and my horse instantly went from fidgety to deeply relaxed. I'm a vibrational medicine pro—this is now my favorite tool."

Again, for the most part, animals don't experience the placebo effect the same way humans do. You can't coach a horse into calming down.

When people start sleeping better, everything else starts getting better, too. If you're stuck in anxiety, if you haven't had a good night's sleep in weeks or months or years, PEMF might be your first domino. The one that tips everything else in a positive direction.

■ How to Fit PEMF Into Your Life (Spoiler: It's Easy)

Turn on your PEMF device and put it in your pocket. That's it. You're done!

It's passive. It doesn't interrupt your day. You don't have to block off time or sit still or count anything. And that ease is what makes it so different from almost every other self-regulation practice out there.

How Often Should You Use It?

Here's what we tell people: **Use it 3 to 4 times a week for 30 days.**

If you don't feel a difference by then, it may not be the proper protocol for your body, or you might've misdiagnosed what's going on.

A lot of people who find their way to PEMF are dealing with long-term, chronic pain or anxiety. They've tried everything else. So when they finally get relief, they don't want to stop. And frankly, they don't listen to my "3x a week" recommendation. They're using it *every day*. Sometimes *three times a day*. And that's fine because it's that easy.

I'll be honest: we still don't know exactly what the long-term "maintenance" dose should be. There aren't large-scale, long-term studies showing whether going from daily use to twice-a-week keeps the benefits going. Everyone's different.

But I will say this: the Earth puts out electromagnetic fields 24/7. Every living thing on the planet is bathed in it. So when people ask me about the long-term effects of PEMF, I remind them— you're already living in it. If it were dangerous, we'd know by now. It's been around for billions of years.

Honestly, I've tried other wellness tools. One of them requires me to sit still for 30 minutes and listen to guided meditations. The guy's voice drives me up the wall. I can only tolerate the sessions without the voice, and those are like 2% of what's on there. So it sits on my shelf.

My wife called it the moment I bought it: *"You'll never use that."*

She was right.

But I use PEMF often because I don't have to *do* anything. It fits into my routine without asking for anything in return.

If you're managing chronic anxiety, the key is just to develop a simple habit:

- Run a protocol at lunchtime.
- Set a reminder to use it in the early evening.
- For sleep, use it one hour before bed and see how it helps you wind down.

■ *Final Thoughts: If Your Pizza Got Hot, It Worked*

Yes, PEMF is invisible. You can't smell it. You can't taste it. You don't feel a jolt like a TENS unit. So, how can it be effective?

We live in a world full of things we use every day without understanding how they work.

Think about the Hubble Space Telescope. Or the James Webb. We're looking at galaxies so far away we don't even have the language for what we're seeing. We're finding things that look like blueberries on distant moons.

And don't even get me started on consciousness. Try sitting down with your smartest friends and defining that. Or anesthesia—how is it that they can knock you out, move your organs around, and you wake up with no memory of it? My wife still thinks that's the wildest part of surgery.

There are mysteries in every direction—from the tiniest subatomic particles to the deepest emotions in your heart. And sometimes, the most beautiful puzzles are living *right inside you*. We don't have to understand every detail to believe something works.

Now and then, I get a doctor—hardcore left-brain, data-only kind of guy—who says, *"We can't use PEMF unless you tell me exactly how it works."*

I say, *"You don't know how aspirin works either."* *Well you* **think** *you do, but it has never been proven"*

Aspirin's been around for 3,000 years, and nobody fully understands the exact mechanism of action. You've got theories, but no real proof. And that's true of almost every drug on the market.

■ The Microwave Pizza Test

Let me wrap up with this: Have you ever heated up a slice of pizza in a microwave?

Of course you have. Everybody has. But **do you know how the microwave heats the pizza?** Most people don't. The theory is that the frequency of the microwave causes water molecules to spin on their axis, generating heat through rotation and friction. But no one has ever actually photographed or videoed a spinning water molecule. Not once. Not ever. There's no tech for that yet.

And you know what?

Your pizza still got hot.

You don't need a lab-grade explanation to believe in what *works*. You use your microwave every day. You don't understand it, but you trust it because the results speak for themselves.

It's the same with PEMF. You may not feel it. You may not fully understand it. But when the anxiety eases, when the sleep deepens, when the pain fades—**that's your pizza getting hot.**

And that's all the proof most people ever really need.

KEY TAKEAWAYS

- Your body runs on cellular electricity, and PEMF recharges those tiny batteries, helping your cells absorb nutrients, eliminate waste, and function better, especially if you're anxious, in pain, or stuck in survival mode.

- PEMF stimulates the vagus nerve and boosts ATP production by up to 500%, creating a ripple effect that calms the nervous system, tones the brain, and trains your body to find its natural rhythm again.

- Results often show up in ways you can see and feel—deeper sleep, less pain, calmer energy—even if the therapy itself feels like nothing at all; the most powerful shifts happen silently.

- Because it's passive and easy to use, people actually stick with it, which means they get real, lasting results without disrupting their routine.

- You don't need to understand exactly *how* PEMF works to believe in it, just like you trust your microwave even if you've never seen a spinning water molecule; when your "pizza gets hot," you know it's working.

CHAPTER FIVE

The Cost of Staying Stuck

Ignoring anxiety means living reactively rather than intentionally. You wake up every day in quiet panic, but you've gotten so used to it, you don't even notice anymore. Roy H. Williams—one of my favorite thinkers—has a line I've borrowed many times: *"Urgent things are rarely important. Important things are rarely urgent."* Most of us live in reverse. We chase what feels urgent, and we call that normal. But "normal" is just a quiet state of panic.

You don't realize how much it's costing you until something breaks. That's when the bill for all those anxious days comes due.

I've always liked the idea that significant life changes are portals—doors we walk through into the next phase of our lives. At the Wizard Academy, we talk about that all the time. And the truth is, addressing your anxiety is one of those doors.

It doesn't have to be some big, dramatic moment, either. Sometimes, all you need is what Matt Damon calls in *We Bought a Zoo*, **"20 seconds of insane courage."** Twenty seconds of just embarrassing bravery. That's all it took for his character to walk up and talk to the woman who became his wife. And, as he said, *"I promise you something great will come of it."*

Think about that for a second—what if everything you want is on the other side of 20 seconds of courage?

I've had those moments myself. My first big public speaking event was in front of 500 people at an Air Force base. I was up all night puking, scared to death. I thought seriously about calling in sick. But I forced myself to go.

And nobody killed me. Nobody even booed. It wasn't that big a deal. But if I hadn't done it, I'd have been stuck in "stage fright" forever. That one moment taught me that staying stuck is often just a matter of refusing to endure 20 seconds of discomfort.

Roy H. Williams jokes about his own anxiety all the time. He says he's kept his car keys in his pocket for 40 years, just in case he needs to bolt out the door during any presentation. That's how deep-rooted this stuff can be. But even he knows you can't let it stop you from stepping through the doors that matter.

Mark Twain nailed it when he said, *"I've been through some terrible things in my life, some of which actually happened."* Anxiety convinces you to live as if the worst-case scenario is already true. You start saying no to new adventures because of some vague, uneasy feeling. You stop pursuing meaningful dreams because deep down, you're convinced you'll fail. And the price of staying stuck keeps rising:

- Your sleep quality drops.
- Physical symptoms show up—digestive issues, chronic pain, headaches.
- Your sense of wonder and curiosity about life slowly erodes. Albert Einstein said, *"The most beautiful thing we can experience is the mysterious. It is the source of all true art and all science."*

One of the most heartbreaking costs of untreated anxiety is what it does to your relationships. I've seen it over and over, and it usually shows up as divorce, or at least the threat of it.

I've got a good friend whose wife's number one complaint is simple: *"He doesn't want to do anything anymore."* And she's right. His anxiety has him trapped. He's got all my devices—I keep telling him to use them—but when anxiety has its grip on you, even taking that first step feels impossible.

It's not just about marriage, either. People start pulling away from everything. They stop socializing. They skip family gatherings. They don't spend time with friends. Slowly, they unplug from the very things that make life feel alive and connected.

If you stay stuck, you lose more than sleep and optimal health. You wash away the adventure of life itself with the people you love, which, in my opinion, is the biggest risk of all.

■ *Why "Pushing Through It" Is So Dangerous*

Pushing through anxiety is like ignoring a smoke alarm. Maybe you don't see the fire yet, but the alarm's going off for a reason.

A lot of us grew up with that tough-it-out mentality. Parents say, *"We walked uphill both ways in the snow, so you can get over it."* You've heard it. Maybe you've said it yourself. But fighting through chronic anxiety keeps you in constant fight-or-flight mode. And in that state, your body can't shift into parasympathetic mode—the "rest and repair" mode you need to heal. You start throwing off your hormonal balance. And if you want to geek out for a second (you know me, I'm going to geek out), it goes all the way down to the mitochondrial level.

Persistent stress actually hampers your mitochondria's efficiency. That's your cell's power plant, its battery. Anxiety drains it, reduces energy production, and ramps up oxidative stress. It even impairs your body's detox system. So no, it's not just "in your head." This stuff shows up in your biology.

We were going to run specific lab tests to prove that PEMF works at the mitochondrial level. But the FDA told me flat out: *"If you prove it changes mitochondria, that makes it a Class I medical device. Millions of dollars. Years and years of research."*

I laughed and said, *"So by your definition, breathing air and meditating are Class I medical devices?"* They didn't think it was funny. But that's how real this is. Chronic anxiety changes you at the cellular level.

The Toughest People Break, Too

I want to share a story that still brings a smile to my face. A friend of mine—Dr. H., an MD deeply involved in this field, told me about a huge man who walked into her office. This guy was six-foot-six, maybe six-eight. A Green Beret. Total badass. And the first words out of his mouth were, *"Whatever you do, don't treat me for PTSD or anxiety. That stuff isn't real. Do something else."*

She said okay. She treated him. Thirty days later, he came back, grabbed her hands, and said, *"Did you treat me for PTSD and anxiety?"*

She smiled and said, *"Yep."*

And this giant Green Beret—who had spent his entire life being tough, fighting through everything—looked her straight in the eyes and said, *"Spend the rest of your life making sure every soldier has one of these devices."*

That's how big the shift was for him. Thirty days. One treatment protocol. And he went from denying anxiety even existed to realizing he had been living in a different world once his brain calmed down.

Even the toughest people crack under the weight of anxiety. Pretending you're fine doesn't make you fine. It just traps you in a burning building.

■ *The Hustle Trap*

Our culture celebrates being busy. We idolize hustle. We give gold stars to the person who's "always on," who "gets shit done." I just read a book titled *Get Shit Done*. That's where we are as a culture.

Corporations love the employees who never ask for help, who grind it out. And society repeats these mantras, such as "tough it out" and "fake it till you make it," as if they are badges of honor.

The dark side of that hustle often means you're ignoring that smoke alarm going off in your head. And because of the stigma, you're too embarrassed to admit it. PTSD? Anxiety? Culturally, we've treated those as weaknesses, not as what they really are—signals from your nervous system that something needs to change.

And because we often confuse constant busyness with purpose, stillness can feel threatening. Trust me, I get this one on a personal level. I caught myself the other day trying to bang out one more email a minute before getting on a call. I had to stop myself.

So if that hustle culture mindset has consumed you, you're not alone. But you've got to ask yourself—are you really winning by running yourself into the ground?

Slowing Down Is Courage, Not Weakness

Many people believe that slowing down to heal is a sign of weakness. I disagree. **Slowing down is the ultimate act of courage.** Healing takes vulnerability. It takes being honest with yourself. At the Wizard Academy, we teach this about sales all the time: *to be likable, you have to be vulnerable.* People do business with people they trust, and trust requires honesty.

The same is true for healing. Slowing down isn't "giving up." It's building a solid foundation so you can grow stronger and live a better life. The strongest people aren't the ones who never stop moving; they're the ones who know when to rest, when to recalibrate, and when to take those 20 seconds of insane courage to step through a new door.

Let's look at some famous examples. Take Simone Biles, one of the greatest gymnasts of all time. She withdrew from the Tokyo Olympics, right in the middle of it all, to protect her mental health. She said, *"I have to focus on my mental health and not jeopardize my health and well-being."* That's courage. But it also shows how far gone she was before she finally stopped.

Or look at Lady Gaga. She's been open about struggling with chronic pain, PTSD, and anxiety. She admitted, *"I was so overworked and in pain that I was like, 'I'm going to die.' I didn't think I'd make it."* Pushing through it only leads directly to a breaking point.

And then there's Prince Harry. He's talked about how his anxiety and panic attacks in his twenties were tied to shutting down his emotions after his mom died. He said, *"I can safely say that losing my mum at the age of 12 and therefore shutting down all of my emotions for the last 20 years has had quite a serious impact on my life."*

Anxiety doesn't care how talented, wealthy, or successful you are—it'll take you down just the same if you ignore it long enough.

■ *Standing on the Edge of Change*

If you're at a crossroads right now—afraid to move forward but also afraid to stay stuck—I want you to hear this: there's no shame in being scared. Fear is simply a signal that you're standing on the edge of change.

I'm a hot air balloonist, and when people tell me they're afraid of heights, I laugh and say, *"Good. You should be."* Every sane person is afraid of heights, at least a little. If you're not, something's probably wrong with you, and honestly, I don't want you in my basket.

But most people imagine a hot air balloon will swing around like a carnival ride. It doesn't. Once you're up there, you're moving at the same speed as the wind. It's calm. Peaceful. Almost magical. The fear is all in the moments before you step into the basket.

Anxiety works the same way. It's the fear of the unknown. But that fear is also your body's way of saying, *"Something is about to happen. Something is about to change."* And change—if you let it—can open the door to a better life.

You are not alone in this. Anxiety is the number one ailment in the world, so there's an entire army of us standing right where you are right now, facing the same door.

So take the next step.

And if you need a little push, go back to Mark Twain's wisdom from the top of the chapter: *"I've been through some terrible things in my life, some of which actually happened."*

Most of what you're afraid of will never happen. Don't let imagined disasters keep you frozen in fear. You deserve more than just survival. You deserve a brilliant, vibrant, meaningful life.

KEY TAKEAWAYS

- Staying stuck costs you more than you realize—your sleep, your health, your relationships, and the adventure of life itself slowly slip away while you convince yourself you're "fine."
- Pushing through anxiety is like ignoring a smoke alarm. Chronic stress rewires you at the cellular level and keeps you trapped in fight-or-flight mode.
- Even the toughest people break. Real courage is slowing down, being honest with yourself, and taking that first vulnerable step toward healing.
- Fear is simply a signal that you're standing on the edge of change. Most of what you're afraid of will never happen, and everything you want might be on the other side of 20 seconds of courage.
- You deserve more than survival. Don't let imagined disasters keep you stuck when a better, more vibrant life is waiting on the other side of that door.

PART THREE

Make Room For Joy

CHAPTER SIX

How to Build a PEMF-Based Calm Practice

We've talked a lot about the science, the theory, and the background of PEMF. That's all important because I wanted you to understand *why* this works before you jumped in. We are now moving beyond theory. This is where you actually go do it.

In the last chapter, I discussed portals—doors we step through to transition into a new phase of our lives. Well, this is one of those doors; it's right in front of you, and it's easier than you think. Access to portable PEMF is here now. It's non-invasive. It fits in your pocket. No office visits. No scheduling appointments at a spa to lie on some giant mat. You don't need to carve out half your day just to calm your nervous system.

And let me say this again because it's that important: **calm isn't a luxury.** It's not some nice-to-have. It's a prerequisite for joy, presence, creativity, and healing. At the cellular level, you can't even *start* to heal until you get the anxiety out of your system. Until you get proper vagus nerve tone, your body won't shift into real repair mode.

If you want to know why I take this seriously, for me, PEMF started as a way to manage sleep, because without it, I'd have brutal nightmares. I'm talking full-on, people-are-trying-to-kill-me kind of nightmares. When I forget to run the device before bed, those nightmares can come back. However, when I run the **Sleep** protocol or the **Brainwave Delta** program, I experience peaceful, dreamless sleep most nights. That alone has been life-changing for me.

Here's what my ritual looks like: most nights—not every single one, but most—I run the Sleep protocol for about 45 minutes to an hour before bed. Then, in the last 15 minutes before I go to sleep, I switch to Brainwave Delta.

I've also always struggled with meditation. Maybe you can relate. Before PEMF, I could focus for about four seconds—seriously, four seconds—before my brain would go full-on monkey brain. Whatever random thought popped in, I was gone. I'm not perfect now, but PEMF has helped me a lot. I can settle into meditation way better than before. It's like PEMF quiets that mental noise long enough for me to actually *be* still, even if just for a little while.

■ *The Simplest, No-Pressure Way to Try PEMF*

PEMF is effortless. You're not committing to some giant routine. You're not hauling yourself to the gym, booking spa sessions, or sitting in a doctor's office. You can do this at home while watching TV, reading, cooking, or even working on your computer.

And here's the best part: you'll know within 30 days whether it's working for you or not. Sometimes you'll know much sooner. I've seen people notice changes right away—things like asthma relief, reduced back pain, or sudden improvements in deep sleep. But if it hasn't worked for you in 30 days, one of two things is going on:

- It's not going to work for you for whatever reason.
- You're running the wrong protocol because you've misdiagnosed what you really need.

Either way, you're not wasting months of your life trying to guess. That's what makes this technology awesome—it's low risk, non-invasive, and you get answers fast.

The "Power of Four" Approach

Currently, we're encouraging individuals in anxiety studies to follow something I call **The Power of Four**. It's still evolving as we learn more, but it's already making a big difference.

The four protocols are:

- **Anxiety Protocol**
- **Relax and Balance**
- **Vagus Nerve**
- **PTSD**

What we're seeing is that everyone's different. Some people get great results from one single protocol. Others find the magic in combining two or more. That's why I recommend trying all four, mixing and matching them, and seeing what works best for you.

■ *Common Beginner Mistakes (And How to Avoid Them)*

You'd think using PEMF would be foolproof—it's intuitive, like an old Apple iPod. Power up, select the protocol, and click play. But **the number one mistake people make is not watching the instruction video.** It's six minutes. Yet every day we get 200 emails asking the same questions that are all answered in that video. So, nicely as I can say this… **watch the video.**

The Power-Level Problem

The second most common mistake is with the power level. The device's screen enters sleep mode after 15 seconds to conserve battery, but the protocol continues to run. People click any button to wake it up and check the time status, so they start pressing buttons and accidentally turn the power way down.

Then they email us saying, "It's not working." Well, yeah, not if you've got it running at level 0 instead of 10.

We're actually adding a message to the next batch of devices that will say: *"Hey, you've turned the power down from 10. Did you mean to do this?"*

And Please... Stop Dropping It in the Toilet

I can't believe I have to say this, but dropping it in the toilet is a common beginner scenario. People will ask me, "How do you know I dropped it in the toilet?" Because it's literally the only way to get it wet.

The device isn't waterproof—it has to "breathe" to function. But we've added water barriers and other protections. If you *do* drop it, grab a blow dryer immediately. We have a whole procedure for that.

Stay Hydrated (No, Coffee Doesn't Count)

Here's another huge one, especially for elderly users: **you need to be hydrated.** Yes, it'll still work if you're not, but it works *better* if you are, especially if you've got electrolytes in your system. Magnesium, in particular, helps PEMF work more effectively.

And don't just *say* you're hydrated. Many people think they are when they're not.

A guy once told me it wasn't working very well for him. I asked, "Are you sure you're hydrated?" He said, "Yes." So I asked, "How much water do you drink in a day?" His answer?

"I don't drink water."

When I pushed, he said, *"Well, I had a protein drink last week."* Another favorite: *"I had three cups of coffee today."*

Newsflash: coffee is the opposite of hydration.

Be Realistic (and Look for the Small Wins)

People often expect dramatic overnight changes. Sometimes, you'll achieve quick wins, such as pain relief or deeper sleep, in a single session. But if you've had chronic mental or physical issues for 20 years, 30 minutes isn't usually going to erase them magically.

Think in terms of cumulative benefits: use it **three to four times a week for 30 days.** That's how you'll know for sure if it's working. And while you're at it, **look for the small wins.**

- Better digestion.
- Clearer thinking.
- Less irritability.

Those small improvements add up.

Track Your Progress (You'll Forget Otherwise)

One of the biggest challenges isn't whether it's working—it's whether you *notice* it's working. People forget how bad they felt 30 days ago. It's human nature. That's why we're building wearable integration into our systems—our own wellness watch is coming soon, but in the meantime, use what you have: a Fitbit, an Apple Watch, an Oura Ring, or a similar device.

If you don't have wearables, keep a diary. Write down how you feel every day. Otherwise, you'll get to day 30 and think, *"I don't feel any different,"* when in reality, you're sleeping better, thinking clearer, and snapping at your spouse a lot less.

The Mindset Mistake

And here's maybe the biggest mistake of all—your mindset.

You've heard of the placebo effect—people get real benefits just because they believe something will work. There's a famous study where a surgeon cut open patients for a knee replacement, but for the control group, they didn't actually replace anything. Those patients still reported almost as much pain relief as the ones who had real surgery.

Well, the **nocebo effect,** as we've discussed previously, is the opposite. If you convince yourself it won't work, there's a reasonable chance it won't. I can almost predict who's going to return the device before they even buy it. They're the ones asking about the warranty and the return policy ten times before they hit "buy." I want to tell them, *"Please, just don't. Save yourself the trouble."*

So **go in with an open mind.** Hope that it helps you. Don't sabotage yourself by deciding ahead of time that it won't.

■ *What a Realistic Daily PEMF Routine Looks Like*

Here's the beauty of PEMF: you don't need to overhaul your life or carve out an hour like you would for the gym. You're already walking around all day with a cellphone in your pocket, right? Well, this is the same thing—except this "phone" is quietly helping you calm your nervous system while you live your life.

A realistic PEMF routine is simple:

- **Use it whenever you think about it.** Keep it somewhere visible so it reminds you to pick it up.
- **Run what you need, when you need it.** If you're trying to sleep, run the Sleep or Brainwave Delta protocols an hour before bed to "jack yourself down."
- **Need energy in the morning?** Run Gamma instead of downing three cups of coffee.
- **If you meditate, run it during meditation.** Tons of feedback says it deepens focus and quiets the mind.
- **Traveling or dealing with anticipatory stress?** Start running protocols days in advance.

One of my favorite examples is horse owners traveling across the country. The *owner* freaks out for a week before even loading the horse, so they should run the anxiety protocol on themselves ahead of time. And for the horse? Run it an hour before the trailer arrives so he's calmer before the stress even starts.

The point is, you don't have to schedule your life around PEMF. Work it into your life, not the other way around.

■ *How Long Before You Notice a Difference?*

Everybody's different, but here's the honest breakdown:

- **Sometimes it's immediate.** Asthma relief, blood pressure drops, and even lower blood sugar levels can occur after just one session. Anxiety often responds quickly, too—many people report feeling calmer in minutes.
- **In our VaguVibe study,** every single person reported reduced anxiety and improved heart rate variability after just one hour.
- **Within 30 days, you'll know for sure.** I've said this before, but if you're not seeing results after three to four sessions a week for 30 days, either you're on the wrong protocol or, for whatever reason, PEMF isn't going to work for you.

For perspective, look at the numbers:

- **PTSD:** 98% success rate within 30 days.
- **Anxiety:** 90%+ success rate using one of the four key protocols (Anxiety, Relax and Balance, Vagus Nerve, or PTSD).

Compare that to drugs, which average about a 60% success rate and come with side effects, risks of dependence, and withdrawals. Nothing is 100%, but PEMF is batting way above average without any of the downsides.

■ *Do You Have to Add Breathwork, Hydration, or Movement?*

The short answer is **no.** Yes, hydration helps. So do magnesium and electrolytes. That's why we recommend drinking a few glasses of water before a session, ideally four glasses in the four hours leading up to it. But don't freak out if you can't. It'll still work; it just works better if you're hydrated. (And, as stated above, coffee doesn't count. Neither does a protein drink you had last week.)

Breathwork and gentle movement can be helpful, but they are not necessary. I don't want people to overthink this or feel like PEMF is one more complicated thing they have to "do right." That's why I dislike devices that require you to sit still for 30 minutes, staring into space, without moving.

The whole point of this technology is that you don't have to do anything special. You can be walking the dog, cooking dinner, answering emails—living your life. Half the time, people forget they're even running a protocol until they notice they suddenly feel better. You'll catch yourself thinking, *"Wait, I'm not as tired. My brain feels clearer. I'm typing faster. I'm actually getting decent ideas."*

So don't overthink it. Just run it.

■ *No Shortcuts*

A lot of people ask, *"Can I just run it for 15 minutes on a stressful day instead of the full session?"* No. It won't work. Here's why:

Each protocol is designed with dozens of frequency pairs—some as many as 76—stacked in a specific order. Your body needs *all* of them. If you cut the session short, you're only giving your body two or three of those pairs, which does almost nothing.

For example, the Sleep protocol runs for 47 minutes, and it's not just looping at the same frequency. It gradually ramps your brain down from beta or gamma (your daytime "amped up" state) to deeper, calmer brainwaves. Quit at 10 minutes, and you're still stuck in beta.

And please don't try to outsmart the system by looping it all night. People ask me that, too. But after a session finishes, it resets to where it assumes you are—your daytime beta or gamma state.

So, if you loop it, you're ramping *back up,* which is the opposite of what you want before going to sleep.

Most protocols are 40 minutes on average; the shortest is 30 minutes, and the longest is approximately two and a half hours. But really, there aren't many things in your life you can't do for 40 minutes with a PEMF device quietly running in your pocket.

■ *Calm Is Not a Personality Trait*

A friend of mine—an ex-Indy race car driver—had been through hell. Four concussions. Set on fire twice. The kind of trauma that rewires your brain and wrecks your sleep.

For over a decade, he was taking *eight* Ambien a night. That's not just bad for you, it's deadly. But he didn't know how else to get any rest.

Then he started using PEMF. He built his own nightly wind-down ritual with the **Sleep** protocol and **Relax and Balance.** Over time, he customized a sequence of brain-balancing and sleep programs that worked for him.

Now he **takes zero Ambien.** And for a guy who was basically killing himself with prescription sleep meds, that's life-changing. That's the power of creating a calm practice.

Calm is not a personality trait—it's a physiological state you can train.

You don't need to "fix yourself" first. You don't need to meditate in a cave or have a perfect morning routine. You don't even need to meditate at all (though PEMF does work great alongside meditation).

Just lead with curiosity rather than control. Put the device in your pocket. Select the protocol you want. That's still my favorite thing about PEMF: it's therapy on the go.

On cross-country trips, one of my friends used to drive 500 miles, sometimes 800 miles out of her way, just to avoid certain bridges. That's how bad her anxiety was. Now she runs the **Anxiety** protocol when she drives, and she told me, *"I see the bridge, and I'm not scared anymore."*

So when you think about it, run the protocol. When you feel the need, run the protocol. Calm isn't magic, but it's close, and PEMF gets you there faster than almost anything else I've seen: **90%+ success rates with most protocols.**

Turn it on. Let it run. Feel the difference.

KEY TAKEAWAYS

- Calm isn't a luxury. It's the foundation for joy, focus, and healing, and PEMF helps you train your body into that calm state.

- Keep it simple: run the right protocols consistently for 30 days, stay hydrated, and look for the small wins that add up.

- Don't overthink it—work PEMF into your life instead of scheduling your life around it; use it while doing everyday things.

- Avoid beginner mistakes: watch the quick-start video, maintain the power level as intended, and allow each session its full run time.

- Calm is trainable, not a personality trait—stay curious, stay consistent, and let the results speak for themselves.

CHAPTER SEVEN

Calm Is the New Normal (And Where Joy Begins)

D ale Carnegie used to say, *"Is it really going to matter in 100 years?"* I can't recall whether it was in *How to Win Friends and Influence People* or another one of his books, but for years, I had to deliberately remind myself of that thought whenever I felt upset or anxious. I'd think, *Okay, in a hundred years, this thing won't even be a blip. So why am I letting it get to me?*

Now, when I'm using PEMF, I don't have to force that thought anymore. I don't have to logic my way into calm. My brain just goes there naturally. It's like my nervous system already knows there's no fire, no tiger chasing me.

Calm is the bridge—the portal—from survival mode into actual living. We've talked about portals before. True joy comes after you've fixed your life, but it *starts* the moment you soothe your nervous system.

Here's what calm looks like in real life: you pause before you react. You breathe before you blurt something out. You give yourself a second instead of snapping. And it's not because you're gritting your teeth and counting to ten. The pause happens automatically.

When you're calm, weird things start to show up in your daily rhythm. You wake up before your alarm clock gently, without the jolt of panic. My wife and I both noticed this. If your alarm's set for seven, you might wake up at 6:58, stretch, take a deep breath, and think about what you want to create today. These changes are subtle, but they're profound. They're the quiet markers that you've crossed into a new normal.

One of my customers, Alex, told me this:

> "*I used to snooze my alarm six times just to avoid the panic waiting on the other side. Now I wake up with music playing, light coming through my curtains, and I actually look forward to the day. It feels like I have my mornings—and my life—back.*"
> — Alex T., former corporate executive

■ *The First Surprises of Calm*

One of the earliest things people notice—sometimes without even realizing it—is that they breathe differently. Deeper. Slower.

And you're not *trying* to do it. Everyone's been told, "Take a deep breath, slow down, relax," but when your nervous system is balanced, your body just does it.

Better sleep is another big one. You wake up rested, not just less tired. The world gets quieter because you are no longer overreacting to it. Your focus sharpens. Your memory improves. You're kinder to yourself and to the people around you.

I noticed this on a recent sailing trip to Belize. We had six family members on a 40-foot boat in super close quarters. In the past, there would've been at least a little snapping or raised voices. This time, we all had a VIBE or a VaguVibe, and there was no fighting, no tension.

When your nervous system calms down, everyday life starts to feel a little magical. I have an aquarium in my office, and in the morning, the sun comes through the glass, bounces off the water, and throws a rainbow across the house. It's such a small thing, but I notice it now. I take the time to appreciate it.

Most people tell me they struggle to describe what PEMF has done for them. They say things like, *"I don't know... something's different,"* and sometimes they even say it with a bit of hesitation, like maybe it's a bad thing. But it's not—it's just unfamiliar. When you've been tense or in pain for years, your body gets used to it. Calm feels so different that you almost don't know how to name it.

> *"I didn't know what I didn't know was missing—until the anxiety lifted and I felt peace for the first time. It wasn't loud or dramatic, just a quiet, steady sense of this is how life is meant to feel. I used to think constant tension was normal, but now I know calm is my natural state."*
> — Rachel M.

Signs Your Focus and Presence Are Improving

When your nervous system calms down, the way you use your time changes. For one thing, your phone starts taking more vacations. You're not compulsively checking it every few minutes.

You also start pulling back from things that drain you without adding real value. In my case, I used to open every single order confirmation email my company received. I was excited, sure—but it was also a distraction. I've had to train myself not to open them, as commenting creates an email chain that pulls me away from the big-picture work I can do alone.

Same with social media. I spend a lot of money on Facebook ads, but I'm hardly ever on Facebook. Maybe twice a year for a few minutes, tops. I don't post much personally anymore—it's just a drain. And customer service? I still peek in now and then to keep a pulse on things, but I'm stepping back more and more. There are people who can do it faster and better than I can, and my time is better spent elsewhere.

The shift is this: you spend more time on what truly matters, not just what's urgent. You listen before you speak. You give space for other people to contribute. And maybe the biggest measurement is how your friends and family respond. They'll tell you you're calmer, easier to be around, and less reactive. That's when you'll know it's working.

■ *How Calm Changes Relationships*

You interact differently with the people around you from a place of calm. You recover faster from conflict. You stop assuming the worst. You don't feel like you need to win every argument.

And people notice. Kids mirror our behavior—sometimes in ways we don't even realize. If you're calmer, kinder, more pleasant to be around, they pick that up. My grandniece Lily is a perfect example. My sister used to remind her to say "thank you" constantly. I thought it was a little over the top, but now, at 15, she's more polite than most adults I know. That's the power of consistent modeling.

At work, calm changes the game. You snap less at co-workers. You approach situations with clarity instead of reactivity. In the corporate world, presentation skills can make or break your career. Sometimes the only impression a senior executive has of you is the one time a year you present to them—and that's how they decide if you're worth promoting.

When you're calm, you present with confidence. In my aerospace days, I got the nickname "Mr. Teflon" because nothing rattled me. Any question just bounced right off—not because I was faking it, but because I knew my material inside and out. That kind of presence comes from being prepared, yes, but it's also about nervous system stability. The more confident you are, the better you perform. The better you perform, the more confident you become. It's a self-reinforcing loop.

A calm nervous system takes you out of survival mode and puts you in a place where you can respond from safety, empathy, and clarity. That's where authentic connection happens. It's how you build healthy boundaries and deepen trust in your marriage, with your kids, with your co-workers.

One of the hardest, most courageous things you can do in any relationship is be vulnerable. When you're calm, vulnerability becomes possible. And when you show it, you build trust that lasts.

■ From Managing Stress to Not Having It at All

There's a big difference between "managing" stress and just not having it in the first place. I didn't fully realize that until friends started pointing it out. They'll say things like, *"Back in the day, you would've lost your mind over that."* And they're right. I used to overreact to every little thing. Now, I'm better at figuring out what's actually important and letting go of the rest.

Take my most recent boat trip. You've probably heard the joke that a boat is a hole in the water, surrounded by wood, you pour money into. On boats, my expectation is that *something* will break. When it doesn't, great. When it does, I'm ready for it.

This trip? Nothing broke. We made it home from Belize through Miami to Orlando without a hitch until we landed. That's when a thunderstorm rolled over the airport and lightning struck, shutting everything down. The baggage handlers weren't allowed outside; therefore, no one could get their bags. We stood there for an hour watching the storm and realized it wasn't going to end anytime soon.

The old me would've been in line at the counter, frustrated, maybe even raising my voice at someone who had no control over the weather. Instead, my wife and I decided, *Let's go get a nice dinner and a hotel, and we'll grab the bags in the morning.* Problem solved.

A new baseline allows you to live in a way where stress doesn't even get a foothold.

■ *Building a Life Around Calm and Joy*

A simple way to start building a calm-centered life is to not reach for your phone the second you wake up. Try setting what I call an 8 p.m. digital sunset—a time each night when your "digital world" goes to sleep before you do. If you're used to scrolling until you pass out, it'll feel weird at first. But that space—both at the start and end of your day—gives your nervous system a chance to recalibrate.

Another thing I've done for decades is schedule white space into my week. Back in my 20s, I created an acronym—SIM—and put it on my calendar as a "super important meeting" twice a week for an entire year. Nobody knew what it stood for, and I never told them. But during that hour, I'd disappear and do something completely unrelated to my work.

In the old days, that meant grabbing a random magazine about hair care, cars, travel, anything outside aerospace, and just flipping through it with my antennas up. I'd ask myself: *What here could apply to my business? Is there an ad or a headline I could adapt?* Sometimes it led nowhere. Sometimes it sparked something big.

At Wizard Academy, we do similar "pointless" exercises—like literally putting the lime in the coconut just because we'd all heard the song but never done it. Or hosting a class called "Worthless Bastards," where there's no agenda. You just hang out, share stories, and see what connections happen. It's amazing how much business and creativity come from those unforced, relaxed moments.

> *"My daughter used to say I was always distracted. That crushed me. So I made a new rule: no phone during our drives to school. Now we talk about music, dreams, random things she's learning. That 15-minute window has become the most joyful part of my day. Calm gave me my connection back."*
> — Amira S.

■ *Why Joy Feels Closer When Calm Is Your Default*

Joy is easier to access when you're out of defense mode. When your nervous system is stuck in fight-or-flight, your inner world is loud—full of worry, fear, and self-judgment. There's no room to notice the good stuff. When calm is your baseline, you're present enough to catch the little things—a laugh, a warm cup of coffee, sunlight streaming in the window.

Biologically, what's happening is you're flipping the switch from S for stress (sympathetic) to P for peace (parasympathetic). You're moving from fight-or-flight into relax-and-repair. Your cells leave emergency mode, cortisol drops, and your body starts healing. With a balanced vagus nerve, your body no longer has to "chase" joy.

These days, my own joy comes from places I wouldn't have expected years ago. This whole energy project—whatever label you want to put on it—is hands down the best job I've ever had. I get to help people and pets, and maybe I'll make some money doing it someday. But even if I didn't, the work itself is worth it.

I've never been a micromanager, but I'm lucky enough to have built a team I trust entirely. They're awesome. One of the most joyful experiences I've had lately was giving out bonuses. One woman had only been on the team for two months when I gave her a Christmas bonus. She just sat there and cried. She told me no one had ever given her a Christmas bonus in her life.

That's the stuff that makes me happy—sharing the win. My wife doesn't even know yet, but by the time this book comes out, it'll be public: at the end of the next quarter, we're starting profit sharing. How many companies do that anymore? Almost none. I'm taking a significant chunk of profit and giving it back to the team. My wife asked if I really wanted to do that, but as long as we're making money, I'm all in. I spend a lot of time thinking about how to distribute it fairly—without creating entitlement—and I'm genuinely excited to hand it out.

I'm also delegating more, which is its own form of joy. My teammate Doris now handles all the Facebook haters, so I don't have to wade into that swamp. She's way better at blocking and filtering than I am, and it frees me up to focus on what matters.

And then there's this—writing this book. That's a joy all its own.

■ *Final Thoughts: Apricot Moments*

Calm has a way of opening doors you didn't even know were closed. It makes room for moments you might have rushed past before—like the man who asked me to carry him a cup of ocean water because his brother, dying of cancer, couldn't make it to the shoreline.

It also makes space for the silly stuff that becomes family legend—like the "apricot" safeword we invented on a sailing trip to stop negative talk before it ruined the mood. When my nephew kept going after being "apricoted" twice, his daughter shot back, "Who do you think you are? You're not above apricot!" The whole place erupted in laughter. Those are the kinds of memories calm gives you—the ones that stick.

When calm is your default state, your body stops bracing for impact and starts thriving at the cellular level. Your stress hormones drop. Nerve signals line up in rhythm. Your mitochondria produce steady, reliable energy. The brain's feel-good chemicals— serotonin, dopamine, oxytocin, endorphins—finally have a clear path to do their work. Inflammation eases, your mood lifts, and joy shifts from something you chase to something that arrives, often when you're not even looking for it.

One of my clients put it perfectly:

> *"I didn't realize how much my body was blocking happiness until it stopped bracing for impact. Now joy just slips in—when I'm cooking, walking, even folding laundry—and it feels effortless."*
> — Fred D.

That's the real gift of calm. Not the absence of anxiety, but the presence of joy—woven quietly into the everyday.

KEY TAKEAWAYS

- Calm isn't something you force—it becomes your natural state when your nervous system is balanced, and that shift quietly transforms how you move through life.

- Subtle signs like waking before your alarm, deeper breathing, and better sleep signal that calm has become your new normal.

- When calm takes over, your priorities realign so you stop chasing what's urgent and start showing up fully for what matters most.

- Relationships deepen because you're less reactive, more present, and more open to vulnerability, which builds lasting trust.

- Joy stops being a fleeting escape and turns into something steady and sustainable, woven into the smallest moments of daily life.

CHAPTER EIGHT

What to Do Next: Tools, Resources, and Your First Step Toward Joy

I f you've made it this far, you're probably ready to take action. That's exciting, but it's perhaps a little overwhelming too. How do you know what's safe and what's going to work for you?

My number one rule is simple: don't hurt anybody. That's always been my top priority. We've conducted extensive testing on these devices, examining levels of magnetic fields, frequency ranges, and energy output to ensure their safety. There are industry standards and government guidelines for acceptable levels, and that's the first box you want to check. If a device can't prove safety, it's off the table.

The next big question: does it work? I don't want to sell voodoo, and you shouldn't settle for it either. Our company has about 70 protocols, and while we don't have gold-standard clinical trials for every single one (nobody does), we collect as much data as possible. We're constantly running studies—the largest PEMF study in the world for PTSD, one for diabetes, another for sleep, and one for Alzheimer's is in the works.

When you're looking at any PEMF product, ask: *What data do they actually have? What are their claims based on?* Too often, the origin of these protocols goes back decades—8,000 practitioners experimenting over 35 years—so sometimes we can't can't even trace exactly where a particular frequency pair came from.

The tricky part is that doctors don't usually publish studies; universities do. Doctors are busy treating patients. So, companies like ours have to step up and conduct the studies ourselves, through third-party, independent labs. And if you're comparing suppliers, look closely at how much effort they're putting into proving their stuff works.

Another big factor is practicality. This was one of the main reasons I built these devices: cost, portability, and simplicity. People always ask me, "What's the difference between your device and something like a BEMER mat?" Here's the short version: it's one piece instead of seven, it's way less expensive (think $400 instead of $7,000), and it's incredibly easy to use. I've heard endless complaints about those mats being complicated, and I didn't want that. I wanted something simple: you pick what you need, hit play, put it in your pocket, and go.

PEMF Then vs. Now: A Side-by-Side Comparison		
Feature	PEMF Mat System (Then)	VIBE "Pocket" PEMF (Now)
Retail Price	$7,000	$399
Technology	1990 technology	2023 technology
Gauss Strength	1 Gauss	9 Gauss
Size/Weight	Large, cumbersome mat with multiple components	Half the size of an iPhone SE, only 2.5 oz
Discreet Use	Not discreet	Very discreet (fits in your pocket)
Protocols	None specific to ailments	60 "specific" copyrighted ailment protocols
Portability	Bulky, not travel-friendly	Portable and FAA "air travel friendly"

The last thing you should always consider is customer support. And honestly, this is something I take pride in. We're the only PEMF company I know of that even has a phone number. We're also the only ones who ship same-day (Monday through Friday), and we have real email support.

That may sound like a small thing, but trust me—it makes a huge difference. This is a unique technology, a new thing for most people, and you're going to have questions. The sad truth is that customer support with a lot of PEMF companies really sucks. Ours doesn't, and I can't tell you how much positive feedback we get about that.

So when you're choosing your first PEMF device, keep these in mind: **safety, proven effectiveness, cost, portability, simplicity, and customer support.** Get those right, and you'll have the best chance of making PEMF part of a life-changing routine.

■ *Sharing Your Device*

The funny thing is, you probably won't have to involve your family in PEMF on purpose because they'll do it themselves. I've seen it happen over and over again. Your spouse borrows it. Your kid borrows it. Your neighbor borrows it and "forgets" to bring it back. Next thing you know, you're the one without a device.

People use it on their horse or their dog, and suddenly they realize they're not even using it for themselves anymore. That's when they come back and buy another one. Our two-pack is one of our best sellers. People want a backup, or one that can be charged while the other is in use. More often than not, though, it's because someone else in the household claimed it.

One of our biggest markets is people with dogs and horses. And here's a fun fact: in the U.S., 91% of horse owners also own a dog.

Yet another reason why our two-pack is so popular—one for your horse, one for your dog, and before long, another for yourself.

Just this week, I got a story from a woman who runs a sanctuary. She had three lame horses that could barely walk, let alone gallop. Within a week of using PEMF, all three of them were running around the field. That's the kind of transformation that still amazes me, even after years of working with this technology.

I immediately told her, "Please shoot some video. Give me a testimonial. You could save a whole bunch of horses' lives—or at least make their lives better—if more people could see this." We hear the same thing from rescues, both dog and horse rescues. They reach out all the time because they've seen firsthand how much better the animals do.

Now, people often ask about the placebo effect. With animals, that argument doesn't really hold up. A horse doesn't know what PEMF is. A dog has no idea you're running a protocol. Sure, they know you're trying to help them—they feel your intention—but they don't have the same expectation of results that humans do. So when you see a horse that couldn't walk suddenly running with its tail high, or when you see a wound heal two to three times faster than usual, that's not placebo. That's PEMF.

From there, it ripples through the whole household. If it worked on the horse, people say, "Maybe it'll work for me." Or they see the dog finally calm during a thunderstorm or fireworks—a huge issue for so many pet owners—and wonder what else it could do.

When my wife and I first started this business, she thought the model was flawed. She said, "There aren't any consumables. No supplements, no creams, no pills. So how are you going to get repeat customers?" And the answer turned out to be family, friends, and pets. They create the demand for a second or third unit.

> *"My 12-year-old chocolate lab has horrible arthritis and cloudy eyes. I have been using the arthritis & anti-aging setting for her and her cloudy eyes have cleared up and she is walking so much better along with groaning less. This device is literally life changing and miraculous! It also stopped shingles dead in its tracks on me."*
> — Arlene Lynette M.

> *"My horse is very anxious during shoeings, especially with her hind legs because she has fused hocks...she was still very nervous, yanking her feet away. When she's nervous she also flaps her lips constantly. I put the PEMF on her yesterday while the shoer was here and it was amazing! After a few minutes she stopped flopping her lips and relaxed with her head down! The shoer was able to trim her hind feet with no issues. I highly recommend this device!"*
> — Mindy B.

> *"I keep giving my VIBE away to help others and having to re-purchase. When you see your dog rebound from being sore, like I did, it sold me. Not solicited."*
> — Dave D.

▪ *Sharing Your Results*

One of the things I encourage people to do is share their results—both with us and with others. I'll even guilt people into it sometimes. I'll say, "Look, this just changed your life—helped your PTSD, lowered your blood sugar, gave you peace. Please let us share your story so someone else can have hope, too."

The truth is, your testimony can save someone else's life. That's not an exaggeration. Especially with conditions like PTSD, diabetes, or chronic stress, people need to hear real stories from real people who were skeptical just like them.

And yes, let's talk about skepticism. Men are usually the hardest to convince. Women are far more likely to try something new, and they're often the ones who nudge their husbands to give it a shot. I've heard the same story frequently: a guy saying, "I didn't believe this. I thought it was nonsense. But my wife wouldn't stop nagging me, so I finally tried it—and I was shocked at the difference." That's how the ripple effect starts.

The other piece that helps people stay consistent is community. One place that might surprise you is the comment sections on our Facebook and Instagram ads. We've had thousands of comments. Now, yes, some of them are haters—we've had to block those. But here's what matters: for every negative comment, we get fifty positive ones. People say things like, *"Thank you so much for inventing this technology. This has changed my life."* That's the kind of feedback that keeps people going. It reminds you you're not alone.

By the time you're reading this book, we'll also be offering free wellness coaching—two sessions a week—so you'll have real-time support and guidance. Plus, we'll keep building our library of customer videos and testimonials so you can see for yourself how PEMF is changing lives.

> *"We've been using the VIBE for just a few weeks and it's completely changed our lives… I am already directing all our clients who come through our healing center to get this device as soon as possible. The price is nothing for what you get. You get your life back!"*
> — Jason K.

> *"Absolutely incredible! I suffered with chronic low back pain for 17 years until I got the VIBE! After using it twice, my low back pain was gone along with the pain meds, a pain clinic that made you feel like you were a drug seeker and years of doctor bills. I can't begin to express my gratitude to Resona Health! You're truly miracle workers!"*
> — Wes D.

> *"My wife of 52 years and I both have serious chronic health issues (cardiac and stroke). We have owned and used this awesome device for over a year now and unreservedly recommend it to our friends and workmates. The benefits of the preprogrammed protocols for multiple health challenges are real. The sleep support and brain balancing protocols are also a daily routine for us both. Stress management too! One of the best self-health care items we have purchased. Excellent +++"*
> — Mike D.

■ Taking Ownership of Your Health

Throughout this book, I've gently reminded you that I'm not a doctor. I'm a rocket scientist who happens to work with this technology. So let me say this right away—**do not ever stop doing what your doctor recommends based on something you read in this book. Don't stop taking your medications, don't ignore their advice, and don't go against their orders just because of me.**

What I *will* encourage you to do is take ownership of your health. Do your homework. Explore the possibilities. Reading this book is part of that process.

The reality is that most doctors are 10 to 15 years behind the latest science and technology. Studies show it takes about 15 years for any new medical advancement to make it into mainstream practice—if it ever does. And 99% of new ideas never make it that far.

There's a reason for this. Drug companies almost entirely run continuing education for doctors. And those drug companies don't have any incentive to teach about PEMF or alternative therapies. Their incentive is the opposite: to keep selling drugs. That's why you hear the old joke about drug companies flying doctors to some tropical island for "continuing education." What do they learn? The details of the latest drug on the market.

So when you bring up something like PEMF, don't be surprised if your doctor hasn't heard of it or dismisses it. It's not on their radar because nobody has paid to put it there.

Here's how I think about it when I'm choosing a doctor for myself. I'll ask, "What should my blood pressure be at age 64?" If they answer 115/75 or 120/80, they just failed the interview. Because for someone my age, the real range should be more like 140–150 over 90. That means they're quoting outdated information.

Same with cholesterol. If I ask whether LDL cholesterol is dangerous and they say yes, they're working off twenty-year-old science. That tells me they're not keeping up. If a doctor can't provide me with up-to-date answers on basic health metrics like blood pressure and cholesterol, they're unlikely to be current on PEMF either.

Why You Need to Stay Informed

Twenty years ago, doctors hated the internet. They didn't want patients coming in with research printed off a website, asking questions, because it forced accountability. Patients could finally say, "This study says something different than what you told me."

That's the world we live in now, and it's a good thing. You have access to more information than ever before. Use it. Question. Compare. Keep learning.

No, you shouldn't ignore your doctor. But you also shouldn't hand over complete control of your health to someone who may be quoting outdated data. Take responsibility, do your research, and make informed choices.

■ *Your First Step Toward Joy*

If you're finishing this book today and wondering what to do next, I'll be blunt: **go try it.**

That's it. There's no risk. We offer a 30-day money-back guarantee. Does PEMF work 100% of the time for every single person on the planet? No—nothing does. But the only way you'll ever know is if you try it.

People sometimes call us and say, "I think this is a scam." Well, if it were, you'd call your bank, reverse the charge, and keep the device. So what do you really have to lose? Nothing. What do you have to gain? Potentially everything.

We've talked about that "love letter" blog post I wrote for the Facebook haters that was basically a list of the top 200 or 300 "scams" in history—things that, at the time, sounded like total voodoo but are now so normal you don't think twice about them.

Cell phones? Magical.
MRIs? Magical.
DNA sequencing? CRISPR gene splicing? Absolutely magical.

All of those things seemed impossible, too good to be true, until they weren't. Until they became everyday tools. That's how innovation works. It always looks impossible... right up until it's not.

The best part is **you don't need anyone's permission to start.** Not your doctor's, not your spouse's, not society's. You can take your health into your own hands right now.

Hope is here. Balance is possible. Calm is attainable. Joy is just within reach. Imagine what life can look like on the other side of anxiety. Then stop imagining and take the first step.

KEY TAKEAWAYS

- Look for PEMF devices backed by safety data, real-world results, and simplicity that fits into daily life.

- The most effective technology is easy to use, affordable, and doesn't require a PhD to operate. Our pocket-sized device was built with that in mind.

- You'll likely end up sharing your device with family, pets, and neighbors, not because you planned to, but because results speak louder than words.

- Share your story because your testimony could be the reason someone else finds relief, calm, or even a second chance at joy.

- Don't wait for permission—do your research, question outdated norms, and take ownership of your health starting today.

EPILOGUE

"Joy is not in things; it is in us."
– **Richard Wagner**

Congratulations! You've done something powerful: you've taken the time to slow down, reflect, and open yourself to the possibility of joy as a guiding force in your life. By reading *Go Find Joy*, you have given yourself permission to step into a life filled with more light, gratitude, and meaning.

Through these pages, you've been reminded that joy is not a fleeting luxury, but a renewable resource—something you can cultivate daily, even in the middle of challenges. You now hold a new perspective: that joy is a choice, a practice, and a habit that can transform not only how you feel but how you live.

But here's the truth—too many people will close this book and return to life as usual. They'll let busyness, stress, or doubt crowd out the spark that could have become a flame. Don't let that happen to you. Doing nothing means falling back into the same old patterns that keep joy at arm's length.

Instead, let this be your turning point. Take the next step: commit to weaving joy into your daily rhythm. Whether that's starting your morning with gratitude, making time for the people you love, or simply pausing long enough to notice the beauty around you, the choice is yours.

Here's a simple ladder to guide you:

1. **Pause and Notice** – Each day, take one mindful breath and ask, "Where is joy in this moment?"
2. **Choose a Joy Practice** – Pick one activity (gratitude journal, nature walk, laughter with a friend) and do it consistently.
3. **Support Your Body and Mind** – Try PEMF therapy with the VIBE. It's a gentle, science-based way to restore balance, reduce stress, and open the door to more energy, clarity, and joy.

As you move forward, imagine how your life can expand: deeper relationships, more resilience in the face of struggle, greater creativity, and a lasting sense of peace. Joy isn't the destination—it's the fuel for the journey.

Now that you know where to find it, go claim it. Go live it. Go share it.

Above all else—go find joy.

LEARN MORE ABOUT RESONA HEALTH AND ENERGY THERAPY AT RESONA.HEALTH

ABOUT MARK L. FOX

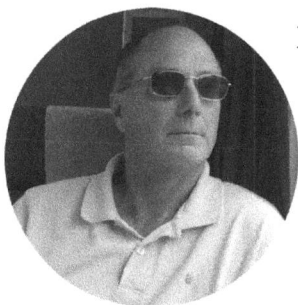

Entrepreneur, scientist, engineer, author, creative thinking consultant, crop formation researcher, and former Space Shuttle Chief Engineer. Hot air balloonist for 35 years, and built his own airplane.

Inventor of VIBE, the world's only "Pocket" Pulsed Electromagnetic Field (PEMF) device. The frequencies are extremely low energy and safe. The VIBE operates at frequencies that are 100,000 times less than your cell phone. The participant simply wears a PEMF device around the neck with a lanyard, or places it in their pocket, while watching TV, reading, walking, cooking, etc.

Resonance Frequency Therapy is for the most common ailments in people and pets. Pain, PTSD, anxiety, sleep, back pain, ADD/ADHD, and 54+ other ailments. No drugs or doctor visits. Therapy in the comfort of your own home.

WHAT MARK'S CLIENTS ARE SAYING...

"Best overall healing device I've purchased in over 27 years... My mother went from needing a walker to walking without pain... macular degeneration improving... this outperforms all my $8,000+ devices.
— *Jason K.*

"After a decade of insomnia post-chemo, I now fall asleep in 5–10 minutes using Brain Wave Delta. Prescription sleep aids didn't help, but this did. It's a miracle."
— *Christine G.*

"My fidgety horse stood still for the first time in his life... head bobbing gone, totally relaxed. Can't wait to try this in the trailer!"
— *Shari B.*

"Low back pain gone after 2 sessions—after 17 years of suffering. No more pain meds or doctor bills. It paid for itself in a month!"
— *Wes D.*

"Immediate relief from fibromyalgia. I wear it in my bra every day. Total game-changer."
— *Cynthia P.*